Kevin R. C. Bard

Thermal Injury

THERMAL INJURY

DONALD P. DRESSLER, M.D.

Associate Clinical Professor of Surgery,
Harvard Medical School,
Boston, Massachusetts;
Surgeon, Mount Auburn Hospital,
Cambridge, Massachusetts

JOSEPH L. HOZID, Ed.D.

Research Associate in Surgery,
Harvard Medical School,
Boston, Massachusetts

PAUL NATHAN, Ph.D.

Director of Cell Biology and Immunology,
Shriner's Burn Institute,
Professor of Physiology (Emeritus),
University of Cincinnati, College of Medicine,
Cincinnati, Ohio

with 37 illustrations

The C. V. Mosby Company

ST. LOUIS · WASHINGTON, D.C. · TORONTO   1988

A TRADITION OF PUBLISHING EXCELLENCE

Vice-president/Publisher: Thomas A. Manning
Project manager: Gayle Patricia May
Manuscript editor: Mary Cusick Drone
Book design: Gail Morey Hudson

Printed in the United States of America

The C.V. Mosby Company
11830 Westline Industrial Drive, St. Louis, Missouri 63146

Library of Congress Cataloging in Publication Data

Dressler, Donald P.
  Thermal injury / Donald P. Dressler, Joseph L. Hozid, Paul Nathan.
    p. cm.
  Includes bibliographies and index.
  ISBN 0-8016-2456-8
  1. Burns and scalds—Treatment. I. Hozid, Joseph L. II. Nathan, Paul. III. Title.
  [DNLM: 1. Burns—therapy.   WO 704 D773T]
RD96.4.D74 1988
617′.1106—dc19
DNLM/DLC
for Library of Congress   87-38318
                                                       CIP

VT/MV/MV 9 8 7 6 5 4 3 2 1

Contributors

FREDERICK B. CLARKE, III, Ph.D.

Benjamin/Clarke Associates,
10605 Concord St., Suite 501,
Kinsington, Maryland

WALTER P. LONG, LIEUTENANT

Rescue Service, Cambridge Fire Department,
Cambridge, Massachusetts

Preface

No affliction of mankind challenges both the patient and the health care professionals as much as that of thermal injury. Although both the overall injury and death rates from fire are decreasing, if there is to be a further reduction in mortality, the health care provider must more systematically address the total care from site of the injury through the initial evaluation and resuscitation phase through all the aspects of wound healing.

The reduction of morbidity is not a new concern; however, when mortality was the main challenge, considerations of morbidity and all of its components were viewed somewhat as a luxury. Fortunately this is no longer the case, and the lessons learned from the care of life-threatening thermal injuries can now be applied to the pervasive lesser injuries. It is readily evident to health care providers that prevention is the most practical solution; e.g., injury from hot liquids can be prevented by design, use, and type of products.

This monograph has been designed to meet the present and emerging needs of health care professionals in the treatment of thermal injury. Given the multiplicity of factors involved, interdisciplinary efforts are required for the development of practical methods for predicting the hazard, preventing the occurrence, rescuing the victims, and treating the patients.

Consistent with the need for providers to extend their knowledge to the fire scene, the first three chapters are concerned with the patterns of fire injury, fire dynamics, fire fighting, and rescue. Chapters 4 through 10 cover the practical, day-to-day clinical applications; and Chapters 11 and 12 address the causes and complications unique to the burn victim and the body areas particularly sensitive to thermal injury.

Chapter 13, Disaster Burn Care, presents a number of new concepts. Catastrophic situations involving thermal injuries were previously viewed as a logistic nightmare; this chapter identifies guidelines for realistic planning for such disasters.

The references have been selected as representative and as a beginning source of information retrieval. It should be noted that, since thermal injury in its many aspects is multidisciplinary, the usual surgical or trauma sources need to be augmented by the behavioral and physical sciences.

In keeping with this multidisciplinary format, we recognize the following contributors: Frederick Clarke, Ph.D., and Lt. Walter P. Long, representing the fire science and fire fighting professions. We would also like to express appreciation to a number of individuals who contributed generously of their time: Eileen Bonner, Col NC USAR (disaster burn care), Costa Chitouras, B.S. (electrical engineering), Dwight G. Geha, M.D. (critical medicine), Varant Hagopian, M.D. (ophthalmology), M. Cherie Haitz, M.S. (library science), John R. Hall, Jr., M.D. (National Fire Protection Association/fire statistics), Merrill C. Johnson, M.D. (nuclear medicine), Lucinda E. O'Loughlin, B.A. (medical records and billing), Ward R. Maier, M.D. (anesthesiology), and Joel Umlas, M.D. (blood banking).

Donald P. Dressler

Contents

CHAPTER

1   Patterns of Fire Injury

MILESTONES

During this century a number of disastrous fires have had a direct impact on social awareness, code enforcement, and medical care. Application of the lessons learned from these catastrophes has significantly lowered the mortality and the morbidity resulting from burns and has had a profound effect on all aspects of prevention.[7,9,15,24]

The 602 deaths that resulted from the Iroquois theater fire in Chicago in 1903 dramatically documented the urgent need for rigorous and enforceable fire codes for public assembly buildings.

Similarly, the deaths of 145 workers in the Triangle Shirtwaist Co. fire in New York City in 1911 highlighted not only grossly inadequate fire codes but also the abysmal plight of the workers, mostly immigrants, in sweatshops where conditions could lead to further large-scale fires and an escalation of thermal injury and mortality.

The 1929 Cleveland Clinic fire, which caused 125 deaths, brought to the attention of the public and the medical profession the hazards of the rapidly emerging synthetic materials. In this case, nitrocellulose in the x-ray film ignited easily and emitted toxic gases.

Unfortunately, the fire in the Ohio State penitentiary in Columbus, Ohio, in 1930, killing 320 inmates, seems to have had little impact on prison fire safety. This problem remains unsolved because of neglect and lack of funding. With the dramatic increase in incarceration sentences, correctional institutions are grossly overcrowded. Given the scale of arson in these institutions, mass casualty care incidents would not be unexpected.

In marked contrast, the Cocoanut Grove fire in Boston in 1942, which killed 492, resulted in the alteration of medical care given burn cases and in the development of new fire codes. These new methods for burn care were immediately implemented in the armed forces in World War II.

In 1944 the Ringling Brothers and Barnum and Bailey Circus fire in Hartford, Conn., in which 168 people died, resulted in new codes, as well as the demise of the circus tents; and the munition depot explosion and fire in Port Chicago, Calif., which killed 300, resulted in new policies for fire control in handling hazardous materials.

Regrettably, fire disasters still occur, especially when fire codes are not uniformly and wisely enforced. Examples can be found in the National Fire Protection Association (NFPA) investigative reports of the Beverly Hills Supper Club fire in Covington, Ky., in 1977, in which 165 people died, and at the Las Vegas MGM Grand Hotel in 1980, in which 65 died.

FIRE LOSS AND INJURY IN THE UNITED STATES
Vital statistics

As reported by the National Safety Council (NSC) of the National Center for Health Statistics, in 1983 the overall burn death rate was 1.8 per 100,000 population.

According to the NFPA, the death rate for urban residential dwellings has remained almost constant for the past 50 years: two deaths per 100,000 population or about 5000 per year.

Fire deaths and injuries by property use

Table 1-1 lists the number of fire deaths and injuries for selected property use in the United States in 1979. Although there has been some reduction during the more recent years, the ratios have remained constant.

Since the fire incidence is higher in the northeast region of the country, which contains many older structures, it will be of interest to note in the coming years whether, with urban renewal and with updated building/fire codes, the deaths and injuries in one- and two-family dwellings will decline and whether commercial buildings such as hotels and industrial properties will be similarly affected by new fire codes.

Table 1-1. Estimate of United States fire deaths and injuries for selected property use categories in 1979 (FEMA)

Property Use	Deaths (%)	Injuries (%)
Residential (total)	5,446 (83.7)	21,100 (69.9)
One- and two-family*	4,175 (64.2)	16,100 (53.3)
Apartments	1,025 (15.7)	3,600 (11.9)
Hotels	165 (2.5)	1,075 (3.6)
Other residential	81 (1.3)	325 (1.1)
Nonresidential	229 (3.5)	3,625 (12.0)
Highway vehicles	650 (10.0)	2,850 (9.4)
Other vehicles	90 (1.4)	1,225 (4.1)
All other categories	90 (1.4)	1,400 (4.6)

From the Federal Emergency Management Agency (FEMA).
*Includes mobile homes.

House fires

Although the largest number of fires result from heating and cooking, followed by arson, and then cigarettes, three fourths of the fire-related deaths result from house fires. There is a variance in incidence between the socioeconomic levels. For example, in fires ignited by heating or electrical equipment in 1984, the number of fires in the lowest-value census tract was nine times higher than in the highest.

Cigarette fires

It is noteworthy that in 1984 the NFPA reported that more than half of the house fires were cigarette ignited. In the United States, cigarette tobacco, unlike pipe and cigar tobacco, is treated with oxidizing chemicals that permit the tobacco to burn hotter, faster, and more evenly. These additives also support combustion; e.g., unlike a pipe or cigar, the cigarette will continue to burn without puffing when enmeshed in upholstery or bedding.

Single fatalities caused by smoking in bed are almost impossible to prevent. However, with the present attitudes toward the health hazards of smoking and the increasing regulations restricting smoking, a substantial decrease in smoking can be expected.

Vehicle fires

Although vehicle fires have been dramatically addressed by Ralph Nader in his book, *Unsafe at Any Speed,* and by the subsequent litigation involving the Ford Pinto fires, the scope, cause, and remedy have yet to be fully elucidated.

In the sunbelt regions, the mobile home has tended to replace the lower socioeconomic residences available in the older cities. The problem of vehicle fires has been compounded by the increase in arson cases and the pervasive problems of highway safety.

Arson

Arson is the fastest growing crime in the country and should be suspected when a building is unexpectedly heavily engulfed in a fire within a relatively short period of time or when multiple ignition sources are suspected. Under these circumstances, the use of an accelerant may result in an unexpected increase in the number of injuries to the firefighters, rescuers, and victims. It is also not infrequent that the arsonist also becomes a victim.

All findings should be accurately recorded for later investigation or prosecution. Any unusual findings should be reported to the authorities. In the event an injury or death occurs as a result of the fire, the arsonist could be charged with assault, intent to murder, or homicide.

Institutional fires

A number of special problem areas relating to institutional fires need to be addressed in more depth. These include fires in hospitals and nursing homes, halfway houses, and correctional institutions. The facilities involved are subject to numerous regulations, and, where enforced through inspection and training, a commendable improvement in the reduction of fire deaths has resulted. Only in facilities that have not been fully sprinkled do deaths occur.

Halfway houses and rooming and lodging houses frequently seem to fall between the cracks of fire code enforcement. Used in many cases by the indigent, homeless, or the recently released mentally retarded or handicapped, they are frequently sites of multiple fire deaths.

Fires in correctional facilities represent a whole different challenge. Not only are the facilities underfunded and overcrowded, but the inmates use fire for attention, revenge, or self-destruction. A review of recent prison fires in Florida, Tennessee, and Nova Scotia gives ample documentation of the problem.

Hot liquid injuries

In a New York study of 156 hot liquid injuries, 50% of patients were under the age of 4, and 27% were over 60 years of age. Of these injuries, 85.2% occurred in the bathtub, 10.7% in the shower, and 4.1% had other causes.[2,6]

Most gas heaters are preset for 140° F (60° C). As noted in Table 1-2, only a 1.5-second exposure at this temperature will result in a second-degree burn, and a 6-second duration will cause a full-thickness injury in adults. For electric heaters the standard is set at 150° F (66° C), which can cause a full-thickness burn in 2 seconds.[22]

Table 1-2. Water temperature vs. time for second-degree burn[24]

Degrees Fahrenheit	Seconds
150	0
140	1.5
130	12
125	42
120	300

The federal standard of 120° F (50° C) in elderly housing and nursing homes can still cause a full-thickness injury to adults in 2 minutes, and in less time to children and the elderly.[7,24] This 2-minute time period is adequate if a person is able to extricate himself promptly; the severely physically or mentally handicapped, however, have difficulty in getting up and over the side of a tub or even out of a shower in 2 minutes.

It is unequivocally distressing to note that parental or guardian abuse, or neglect, is not uncommon in scald burns of children. Guidelines for identifying suspicious cases are detailed in Chapter 11.

TRENDS IN FIRE PREVENTION
Factors affecting life safety

A number of factors must be considered in determining the overall fire hazard and, concomitantly, in developing cost-effective fire protection/prevention measures: structure design; facility use; location; materials; construction; furnishings; adherence to fire codes; and number, physical, and mental condition of occupants. Given its presence in the living space environment, a product's flammability, including ease of ignition and flame spread, and its toxicity are critical considerations in the selection process.[10,11,12]

The box on p. 6 lists the physiological factors affecting survival during a fire. The actual escape response will also depend on the degree of vision, which can be adversely affected by obscuration of the exit signs caused by smoke density and opacity, as well as by physiologic factors such as loss of color and fine vision when the oxygen in the atmosphere falls below 17%.

Training and familiarity are important considerations in ensuring escape and/or survival. It is not uncommon to find victims completely confused in the fire situation. The presence of physically or mentally handicapped people within the structure poses special problems that only forethought, design, and training can overcome. The need for bilingual instructions, exit signs, and even rescue personnel, has often been neglected in the past and should be part of all fire safety programs. Given the prevalence of pets in our society, including their involvement in pet-facilitated therapy for the disabled and elderly, their rescue also requires attention.

Physiological factors affecting survival

Increased carbon monoxide concentration	Direct consumption by fire
High temperatures	Fear
Noxious or toxic gases	Preexisting disease
Smoke	Duration of exposure
Decreased oxygen concentration*	Associated injury

*Actually, life depends on the partial pressure of oxygen, i.e., 160 torr, whereas combustion depends on the percent of oxygen in the atmosphere.

Table 1-3. Trends in fire causes*

Cause	1959 (%)	1972 (%)	1981 (%)
Heating and cooking	22.9	16	42
Smoking and matches	18	12	8
Electrical and appliances	13.9	16	13
Flammable liquids and explosions	6.5	7	1
Open flames and sparks	6	7	4
Lightning	3.3	2	1
Children and matches	3.9	7	5
Incendiary or suspicious	2.3	7	12
Spontaneous ignition	2.6	2	1.2
Miscellaneous, known	14.1	2	5.8
Miscellaneous, unknown	6.5	20	7

*From the Federal Emergency Management Agency (FEMA).

Trends in fire etiology

There have been important trends in fire etiology (Table 1-3), including a reduction in burn injury. Some reductions, such as those from smoking and matches, may reflect increasing public awareness and education, including the use of prevention measures such as flame-retardant materials in children's sleepwear and the selection of approved interior decorator and construction materials.[17,24,28,29]

On the other hand, some of the reduction in burn injury may simply reflect a better reporting system, although improved reporting usually shows an increase.

Building and housing factors

Building/fire codes. It should be noted that present building/fire codes have been highly effective in reducing fire deaths from flame and, concomitantly, from smoke inhalation. When a gross violation occurs, the results are tragic. Examples are readily found when recent hotel fires (e.g., the Beverly Hills Supper Club fire) and various prison fires are reviewed. If the codes had been rigorously enforced, it is doubtful that a large loss of life, or even the fire itself, would have occurred.

Moreover, the devastating recent fires outside the United States such as in the Philippines, South America, and Japan can also be attributed to lack of enforcement of building codes and thus gross deficiencies in them.

Safety construction. Although there have been a number of hotel fires since the MGM Grand catastrophe, including the Dupont Plaza Hotel fire in San Juan, Puerto Rico, in 1987, in which 95 people died, increased code enforcement coupled with the public awareness of the problem have resulted in major improvements in building construction, emphasizing fire prevention and/or capability. For example, the following measures have become standard features of any new building/housing construction: the installation of properly rated smoke alarm detection systems, pressurized stairwells, more extensive use of fire-rated construction materials (e.g., dry wall), and the widespread use of sprinklers. According to the NFPA, there have never been multiple fire deaths in a properly sprinkled building. However, deaths can occur in the room of origin even with sprinklers.[4,24,28]

Smoke detectors

The rapid development in the past decade of inexpensive smoke detectors has supplanted heat detectors, both in cost and early warning, in residential dwellings. In commercial buildings, both smoke and heat detectors are used in a system of early detection.[8]

There are two types of smoke detectors: ionization and photoelectric. The ionization type responds slightly faster than the photoelectric to an open, flaming fire; the photoelectric has a quicker response to a smouldering fire. Either one is acceptable, although the ionization type is now more common.

There are also two types of connections: a single-station battery mode, which has the advantages of ease of installation, low cost, and nondependency on the house power system; and the installation system connected directly to the house power, with switches that are not easily accessible and thus cannot be accidentally turned off. The installation system does not rely on battery replacement, and, more important, it can be installed in series, so that if one detector sounds, all the detectors in the dwelling will also signal. Even if a battery-operated system is the first choice, a dual system is recommended and often required in all new installations.

The recommended locations for smoke detectors are in the hallways outside the bedroom doors; hallways by the living room and dining room, but far enough away from the kitchen so that usual cooking does not set off the alarm; and at the top of the basement stairs. Additional alarms can be added to each bedroom and near the heating system. They should always be placed on the ceiling, or within 4 to 12 inches of the ceiling on a side wall. In ranch and split-level homes, detectors should also be placed within each major section and at each level.

In addition to smoke detectors, training in and planning for emergency procedures such as responding to alarms, feeling the doors for heat before opening, identifying escape and alternate escape routes, establishing a meeting place outside the dwelling, and reviewing procedures for calling the fire department are essential. Each occupant should know the location of other occupants and have emergency lighting. Almost needless to state, smoking in bed is to be condemned.

Special attention should be paid to the sleeping quarters of children and any disabled people in a dwelling unit. These areas should be identified and suitable attention given to escape plans.

Smoke detectors save lives: in the United States and in England, according to NFPA statistics, the risk of death is reduced 50%.

ANALYSIS OF FIRE DEATHS
Overview

What actually causes death or injury during fire? The data are far from complete; but during the past 50 years, according to NFPA information, the number of deaths in this country has decreased from approximately 20,000 in 1933 to 5000 in 1985. And at the same time the population has increased from 110 million to almost 240 million.[7,19,24,32]

To account for this decrease in mortality, several changes should be considered: smoke inhalation has often been stated to be the major cause of death in fires. This statement is misleading. In 50% of fire deaths, the victims arrive at the hospital alive; those that suffer only from smoke inhalation will survive if associated cardiovascular disease, traumatic injuries, drug overdosage, or cutaneous burns are not present. In contrast to previously reported high death rates from shock and burn wound sepsis, the most common cause of pulmonary death in victims of smoke inhalation is pulmonary sepsis. The cause of this high susceptibility to pulmonary infection and death may be related to the inhalation of toxic products, but there are many other reasons such as the presence of cutaneous burns, malnutrition, and dysfunction of the pulmonary host defense mechanisms.

It is important to be aware that a burn injury is not limited either in its deleterious effects to the skin or in inhalation effects to the bronchopulmonary surfaces.

Comparative analysis

Table 1-4 compares the cause of death in burn patients at three different time periods during the past 30 years. Although the data are from my files at two different facilities, the patient groups are similar in age and socioeconomic status. The causes of the injuries were different in that the latter group in California represented fewer

Table 1-4. Comparison of cause of death in three groups of burn patients

Cause of death	1956-1964* (284 patients)	1965-1968* (201 patients)	1980-1981† (286 patients)
Shock	17	7	6
Burn wound sepsis	12	4	5
Respiratory complications	6	20	(13)‡
Myocardial infarction	3	0	3
Carcinoma	1	0	(1)‡
Pulmonary embolus	(9)‡	2	0
Gastrointestinal hemorrhage	(1)*	0	0
Suicide	0	1	(4)‡
Cardiovascular accident	0	2	2
Multiple trauma—homicide	0	0	1
Total deaths	39	36	17
% Mortality	13.7	17.9	5.9

*Boston City Hospital, Boston, Mass.
†San Bernardino County Medical Center, San Bernardino, Calif.
‡Secondary cause of death.

building fires and a slightly greater number of substance abuse situations than in the Boston groups.[35] However, this is representative of the trends throughout the country.

Shock is no longer the major cause of death, but does occur in the massively burned patient. In these patients vigorous resuscitation results in cardiac failure, whereas reduction of fluids contributes to hypovolemia, oliguria, hypotension, and death.

Burn wound sepsis is still the major cause of death in those patients with massive burns in whom the body defense mechanisms are depleted and who then fall prey to any opportunistic bacteria or fungus infections. Death from respiratory complications increased precipitously during the second reported period, 1965 to 1968, after the introduction of effective topical antimicrobial therapy, but before the wide introduction of newly available methods of ventilatory support.

At present, respiratory deaths occasionally occur as a result of adult respiratory distress syndrome (ARDS), but more commonly in those that survive the initial resuscitation period, death is caused by pulmonary sepsis.

Myocardial infarction continues to be a problem and is understandable in view of the stress of the initial injury and the subsequent treatment. Just as with cerebrovascular accidents, death from myocardial infarction will probably increase with the aging population.

Consistent with the generalized trends initiated even before the major improvement in burn care made in the early 1960s, deaths caused by pulmonary embolus and stress ulcers have decreased during the past 30 years.

Although there has always been an awareness that a number of burn victims had psychological problems before their injury, only recently is this being fully appreci-

Table 1-5. Comparison of three groups of burn patients with second- and third-degree burns in relation to mortality and area of burn

Burn area (%)	Deaths/total no. of patients		
	1956-1964*	1965-1968*	1980-1981†
0-29	15/257	9/166	0/218
30-39	6/9	3/8	3/23
40 and over	18/18	24/27	12/39
	$LD_{50} = 26\%$‡	$LD_{50} = 38\%$‡	$LD_{50} = 65\%$‡

*Boston City Hospital, Boston, Mass.
†San Bernardino County Medical Center, San Bernardino, Calif.
‡Percent of total BSA burn at which there is a 50% probability of survival.

ated. In view of this, suicide as a cause of death is being recognized. Similarly, homicide related to the increasing crime of arson is also being noted.[13,14,25,30]

Probit analysis

The mortality rate tabulated in Table 1-4 can be highly misleading, since this simple method does not account for many important variables, most particularly, the varied percentage of total body surface area (BSA) burn within each group.

Table 1-5 uses the probit analysis method introduced by Bull and Fisher in 1954,[4] Pruitt and associates in 1964,[27] and Rittenbury and co-workers in 1965.[31] To analyze burn data, this method factors not only the numbers in each category, but also the percent of TBSA burn. Generally, at least 100 patients with burns severe enough to require hospital admission or with major burn injury are necessary to provide any conclusions concerning treatment trends. These results are similar to those reported from other burn centers during the same time periods with adjustments for type of facility (i.e., community hospital, burn center, tertiary facility) and patient age.

This type of data cannot be used to predict the outcome of an individual patient or that of small numbers of patients, except in general terms. But it is evident that the LD_{50} per percent of TBSA burn has increased considerably during the past 20 years.

Furthermore, it is of more than passing interest to note that in most burn centers a plateau has been reached, with only slight inroads being made into the survival of the more massive burns involving over 65% TBSA, the elderly, or those with other complicating injury or diseases. These data reveal that there is an urgent need to improve early care at the fire site of those persons with major injuries and to make a concentrated effort to reduce the morbidity of the vast number of less seriously burned persons.

Autopsy

It is essential to analyze fire deaths, as well as injuries, to determine cause, to develop preventive measures, and to treat. Adequate burn autopsies are seldom performed, with the cause of death being recorded as fire and/or smoke inhalation.

Even when an autopsy is adequately performed, it is often difficult to describe the sequence of events that led to engulfment by flames, saturation by carbon monoxide, premortem and postmortem increases in blood cyanide levels, or to simply elucidate the panic that results in a failure to escape.

Classification

Occurrence of death by fire can be divided into four phases: (1) in fire, (2) immediately following extrication or admission to a medical facility, usually in a moribund condition, (3) within the first few days as a result of nonrefractory shock or associated injuries or disease, or (4) late, usually caused by overwhelming sepsis from an opportunistic organism.

FIRE FIGHTER AND RESCUE INJURY AND DEATH

Fire fighter and fire rescue injuries are a special concern. The NFPA reported that in 1983 there were 99,300 fire fighter injuries and 117 deaths. These injuries can be acute and consist of cutaneous burns and/or smoke inhalation or often are related to other trauma.[7,20,21,24,33,34,36]

The term "heart lung" diseases refers to the Workman's Compensation Law in most states, wherein it is presumed that any acute "heart lung" occurrence at a fire scene is assumed to be the result of the fire. Although it could be argued that other factors such as preexisting disease, previous exposure, or a cigarette-smoking history may be present, there is no question that the stress inherent at a fire must be at least a major aggravating factor.

According to the NFPA (1981), the actual injury rate per fire was highest in communities of over 500,000 in the Northeast, with 7.1 injuries per 100 fires, and lowest (1.8 injuries per 100 fires) in the smaller western communities.

The most frequent cause of death was trauma (34%); 32.8% were caused by myocardial infarction or heart attacks. Deaths due to drowning were 2.6%, to electrocution 2.6%, to burns 6.9%, to internal trauma 34.5%, and to smoke inhalation 9.5%. As would be expected, trauma was more common in the younger age group, and heart attack in the older fire fighter.[3,5]

There have been a number of studies on fire fighters to evaluate the chronic effects of smoke inhalation. One study, reported by Unger,[37] on 30 fire fighters after severe smoke inhalation, found decrements in both forced expiratory volume (FEV_1)

and forced vital capacity (FVC) with a preserved ratio of FEV_1 to FVC, which is consistent with restrictive ventilation that had persisted at 18 months' follow-up.

Unfortunately, however, there were no preexposure baseline studies. Musk and colleagues[23] and Loke and associates[18] reported similar small-airway obstructive disease, but again the studies had too many variables that were not controlled, and, therefore, the results were not conclusive.

The largest study of fire fighters was in Boston, Mass.[26] Twice the degree of pulmonary function loss anticipated was revealed among 1430 fire fighters studied in 1970, and again in 1972. However, 3- and 6-year follow-ups showed no further loss, which would have been expected with time and/or repeated exposures. Similarly, it would have been expected that fire fighters would have an increased cancer rate due to exposure, but in the limited studies so far, this has not been demonstrated.

Fire fighter injuries can be prevented by periodic physical evaluation, physical conditioning, use of good equipment, particularly self-contained underwater breathing apparatus (SCUBA) gear, training, and, most important, department policies and procedures that emphasize discipline and safety.

REFERENCES

1. Axford, AT, et al: Accidental exposure to iso-cyanate fumes in a group of firemen, Br J Ind Med 33:65, 1976.
2. Baptiste, MS, and Feck, G: Preventing tap water burns, Am J Public Health 70:727, 1980.
3. Barnard, RJ, Gardner, GW, and Diaco, NV: "Ischemic" heart disease in fire fighters with normal coronary arteries, J Occup Med 18:818, 1976.
4. Bull, JP, and Fisher, AJ: A study of mortality in a burn unit: a revised estimate, Ann Surg 139:269, 1954.
5. Dibbs, E, et al: Firefighting and coronary heart disease, Circulation 65:943, 1982.
6. Feldman, KW, Schaller, RT, and Feldman, JA: Tap water scald burns in children, Pediatrics 62:1, 1978.
7. Fire almanac, Quincy, Mass, 1984, National Fire Protection Agency.
8. Hall, JR, Jr: A decade of detectors: measuring the effect, Fire J 79:37, 1985.
9. Jones, JC: A brief look at the hotel fire record, Fire J 75:38, 1981.
10. Karter, MJ, Jr: Fire loss in the United States during 1980, Fire J 75:60, 1981.
11. Karter, MJ, Jr: Fire loss in the United States during 1984, Fire J 79:14, 1985.
12. Kolara, G: Fire! New ways to prevent it, Science 235:281, 1987.
13. Kolman, PBR: The incidence of psychopathology in burned adult patients: a critical review, J Burn Care 4:430, 1983.
14. Layton, TR, and Copeland, CE: Burn suicide, J Burn Care 4:445, 1983.
15. Layton, TR, and Elhauge, ER: US Fire catastrophes of the 20th century, J Burn Care 3:21, 1982.
16. Lefcoe, NM, and Wonnacott, TH: Chronic respiratory disease in four occupational groups, Arch Environ Health 29:143, 1974.
17. Levine, MS, and Radford, EP: Fire victims: medical outcomes and demographic characteristics, Am J Public Health 76:1077, 1977.
18. Loke, J, et al: Acute and chronic effects of fire fighting on pulmonary function, Chest 77:369, 1980.
19. Marshall, WG, Jr, and Dimick, AR: The natural history of major burns with multiple subsystem failure, J Trauma 23:102, 1983.
20. Mastromatteo, E: Mortality in city firemen. I. A review, AMA Arch Ind Health 20:1, 1959.
21. Mastromatteo, E: Mortality in city firemen. II. A study of mortality in firemen of a city fire department, AMA Arch Ind Health 20:55, 1959.
22. Moritz, AR, and Henriques, FC, Jr: Studies of thermal injury. II. The relative importance of time and surface temperature in the causation

of cutaneous burns, Am J Pathol 23:695, 1947.

23. Musk, AW, Peters, JM, and Wegman, DH: Lung function in fire fighters. I. A three-year follow-up of active subjects, Am J Public Health 67:626, 1977.

24. National Fire Protection Association: Fire protection handbook, ed 15, Quincy, Mass, 1981, National Fire Protection Association.

25. Nielsen, JA, Kolman, PBR, and Wachtel, TL: Suicide and parasuicide by burning, J Burn Care 5:335, 1984.

26. Peters, JM, et al: Chronic effect of fire fighting on pulmonary function, N Engl J Med 291:1320, 1974.

27. Pruitt, BA, et al: Mortality in 1,100 consecutive burns treated at a burn unit, Ann Surg 159:396, 1964.

28. Rarig, FJ: Assessing the fire hazard, Fire J 73:34, 1973.

29. Rarig, FJ: The problem of smoke in fires, Plast Polymers 42:168, 1973.

30. Reddish, P, and Blumenfield, M: Psychological reactions in wives of patients with severe burns, J Burn Care 5:388, 1984.

31. Rittenbury, MS, et al: Factors significantly affecting mortality in burned patients, J Trauma 5:587, 1965.

32. Rossignol, AM, et al: Hospitalized burn injuries in Massachusetts: an assessment of incidence and product involvement, Am J Pub Health 76:1341, 1986.

33. Sidor, R, and Peters, JM: Fire fighting and pulmonary function: an epidemiologic study, Am Rev Respir Dis 109:249, 1974.

34. Sidor, R, and Peters, JM: Prevalence of chronic non-specific respiratory disease in firefighters, Am Rev Respir Dis 109:255, 1974.

35. Silverstein, P, and Dressler, DP: Effect of current therapy on burn mortality, Ann Surg 171:124, 1970.

36. Stewart, RD, et al: Rapid estimations of carboxyhemoglobin level in fire fighters, JAMA 235:390, 1976.

37. Unger, KM, et al: Smoke inhalation in firemen, Thorax 35:838, 1980.

2 The Fire Problem

Burning process
    Components of smoke
    Measurement of smoke toxicity
    Burning behavior of materials
    Assessment of fire hazard
Fire fighting and rescue
    Building hazards
      Type of use
      Type of construction
      Building height
      Fire site accessibility
      Floor load
      Construction hazards
    Response context
      Time and day
      Climatic conditions
        Temperature
        Storms
    Fire dynamics
      Type, duration, and progress of fire
      Conditions of stairways and fire
        escapes
      Presence of smoke or heat alarms
        and systems

    Presence of wet or dry sprinklers
    Illumination
Personnel
    Number and proficiency of fire or
      rescue personnel
      Staffing
      Specialized training
      Weather conditions
    Familiarization with building
    Knowledge of location and numbers
      of occupants
    Availability of public utility personnel
Equipment
    Amount and type of fire fighting and
      rescue equipment
    SCUBA equipment
    Other specialized equipment
Occupant hazards
    Number and location
    Special population groups
    Physical condition and behavior of
      occupants
    Language barriers

BURNING PROCESS*

A flame burning over a liquid or solid surface is a familiar sight to everyone. A close look at the phenomenon involved, however, reveals that it is a highly complex process. Flaming combustion occurs in the vapor phase. Hence, for ignition to occur, the fuel must be heated to a degree that fuel vapor begins to escape from its surface, and does so at a rate sufficient to form a flammable mixture with the air above it. If this condition is reached and if the mixture is hot enough to ignite, ignition will

*Contributed by Frederic Clarke, Ph.D.

occur. Most of the heat from the flame is carried off by the hot gases produced, but some of it is returned to the fuel surface beneath the flame by means of radiation. This radiant heat vaporizes more of the fuel, and the fuel vapor rises and burns as it mixes with air and enters the hot flame.[4,5,6,10]

A similar mechanism explains how a fire spreads. Unburned material adjacent to the flame is heated by radiation from the flame. A flame almost always spreads upward much more readily than it spreads horizontally or downward. This is simply because the buoyant hot gases produced by the flame rise, so that the unburned material located above the flame receives not only radiation but additional energy from convected gases as well. More energy delivered to the unburned fuel surface causes the surface to heat up more quickly, and, correspondingly, the flame spreads faster.

The usual measure of a fire's size is its intensity, i.e., the quantity of power, or energy per second, produced.[6,7] The actual chemical reactions between the fuel and air occur almost instantaneously, and the rate at which the fuel reaches the flame is usually slow by comparison, so that the fuel reacts as soon as it arrives. Thus the speed at which energy is released, i.e., the intensity with which the fire burns, is a function of the rate at which the fuel vaporizes. This explains why a pan of gasoline burns more vigorously than a slab of polyethylene of the same surface area and weight, even though the two produce about the same overall energy on combustion. Less energy is required to vaporize a given amount of gasoline than to vaporize the polyethylene, which must be chemically decomposed before it forms any volatile fragments; thus a given amount of energy radiated back from the flame produces more fuel to burn in the case of gasoline than it does in the case of polyethylene.

The essential physical phenomena of the burning process are illustrated schematically in Fig. 2-1. The fuel bed below the flame is vaporized; and the combustible fuel vapor enters the flame, mixes with air, and burns. The expanding thermally buoyant gases produced rise as they burn. This rising column of hot gas, called the fire plume, entrains air through the expansion and turbulence created by the burning process. If sufficient space were available, the hot gases would continue to rise and mix with more air until the combination of expansion, mixing with air, and radiant cooling had reduced them to the same temperature as the surroundings, at which point the fire gases would rise no further. However, most fires that are threats to humans occur in buildings, and the result of a fire burning in a normal-sized room is generally that the hot gases rise toward the ceiling, are contained by the ceiling, and begin to bank downward, filling the room much like an inverted bathtub. When the hot gases have descended to the level of the top of an open door or window, they spill out of the room into adjacent areas. Fig. 2-2 shows the steady burning of a chair, or some similar-sized object, in a typical room. The air originally contained in the room will only support combustion for a few seconds, and additional air must soon be supplied through the doorway or windows. The same vents serve to exhaust the hot smoke at the top as cool air comes in the bottom. A steadily burning fire thus serves

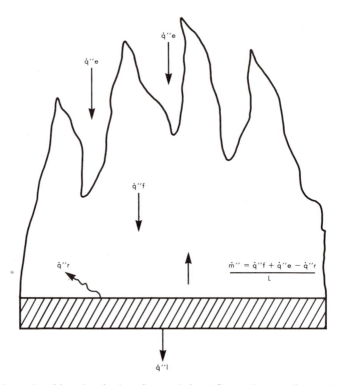

Fig. 2-1. Schematic of burning fuel surface. $\dot{q}''$, heat flux; $\dot{m}''$, mass loss rate; L, effective heat of vaporization. *Subscripts: e,* external (e.g., rest of room or imposed as part of a test method); *f,* from flame itself; *r,* reradiated from fuel; *l,* lost to interior of fuel or to surroundings.

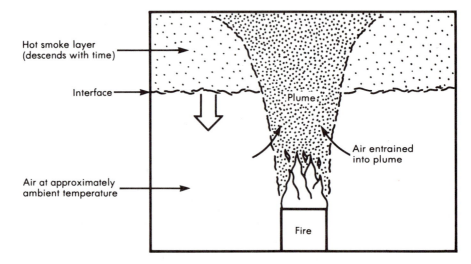

Fig. 2-2. Schematic of fire phenomena.

effectively as a pump to draw cold air into the room, react it with the fuel or mix it with the products of combustion, and exhaust it into the upper level of the room and out the vent.

In most modern offices or residences, there is enough fuel available that the air supply eventually becomes the limiting reagent in the combustion process. This means that the size of the fire is limited by the rate at which the air can enter the room through the vents, keeping in mind that the same vents must also exhaust the smoke. A hot upper layer rapidly develops, which acts on the ceilings, the walls, the floor above, and later on the floor below, as well as on the furnishings. If these materials are also combustible, additional fuel vapor is eventually supplied, not only in the vicinity of the flame, but throughout the room wherever the radiant energy strikes a combustible surface. Eventually, there will be sufficient combustible vapor throughout the room so that burning is no longer confined to the original fuel bed. This phenomenon, called full room involvement or "flashover," is usually the transition point between a fire being confined to the room of origin and its leaving that room to involve adjacent rooms and, eventually, the rest of the structure.[4,12]

Combating a fire is much easier if it can be done before flashover is reached. This is because the delocalized burning makes it difficult to know where to apply a limited amount of water, and the presence of large amounts of heat and flame well away from the initial fire source means that the fire is difficult to approach closely enough to effect extinguishment. Generally speaking, normal offices and residences have rooms that are small enough and contain enough fuel so that flashover can be expected if the fire is allowed to burn unchecked. Once room flashover has occurred, the rest of a typical dwelling, e.g., a floor of a house, or an apartment, can be expected to become involved in a matter of a very few minutes. Flashed over rooms generally provide heat outputs of several megawatts, and fires of this size are extremely dangerous. At flashover, human life will have become untenable. The temperatures in the room at this point exceed 900° F (500° C), and carbon monoxide levels in the smoke will be of the order of 5% to 10%, or 50,000 to 100,000 ppm.

The actual agents of hazard from a fire depend on where a victim is in relation to the fire, as well as the detailed circumstances of burning, i.e., the fire scenario. Both the heat from the fire and the smoke are threats, the relative effects of which will be discussed further in the following sections. First, however, it is important to understand the nature of smoke.

Components of smoke

In this discussion smoke is intended to mean the totality of combustion products, whether gaseous, liquid, or solid. Operational distinctions among soot, the gaseous products of combustion, and any incompletely burned materials that appear as aerosols are of little importance, since they are transported and inhaled together. In large buildings there may be some separation of the soot and aerosols from the fire gases after the smoke has flowed through many cracks or around corners or similar obstacles. However, in general, it is more convenient to characterize the entire complex mixture simply as "smoke." The typical gaseous components of smoke are carbon monoxide, carbon dioxide, and water vapor. If the burning material contains nitrogen, there may be small amounts of hydrogen cyanide, oxides of nitrogen, or ammonia present. If the fuel contains sulfur or halogens, sulfur dioxide or hydrogen halide gas can generally be expected in the smoke.[1,3,8,11,13]

Only a very small number of fuels, however, burn totally to gaseous products. Some of the opacity of smoke is caused by water vapor, which is originally produced in the gaseous state but cools as the smoke gets farther from the fire to produce a visible cloud. In addition, most burning organic materials produce some finely divided carbonaceous material, or soot. The sooting tendencies of materials differ appreciably and, moreover, depend on the amount of air available. In addition to obscuring light, the soot often serves to carry with it other combustion products absorbed on its surface such as partially burnt hydrocarbons and pyrolysis products that are not readily burned (such as hydrogen chloride). These products also appear in the smoke in relatively free form. As the smoke gets farther from the fire and cools a bit, products that are initially gaseous may condense to form aerosols. Gases that are hydroscopic such as hydrogen chloride can be expected to combine with the water vapor in the smoke to yield an aerosol of the corresponding mineral acid.

Obviously, the diffusion properties of a relatively large aerosol particle are substantially different from those of a gas such as carbon monoxide. However, the smoke is generally propelled by the thermal buoyancy from the fire, and the differential diffusion of the various components is very small by comparison. This is why it is usually sufficient to regard smoke as an intimate mixture of all of its various components, except in special cases.

The simplest way to measure a material's tendency to smoke is by its "mass optical density," which is the amount of light-obscuring power produced by the smoke from a unit weight of burned material. The mass optical densities for most common materials lie within approximately a fivefold range. Fuels derived from aromatic hydrocarbons such as kerosene or polystyrene are inherently more smoky than those derived from cellulosics such as wood. However, the presence of additives and the conditions under which the materials burn can often overshadow, or change, the relative smoking characteristics of materials. In practice, the amount of smoke produced in a given time is a product of the mass optical density of a material and its burning rate. Both of these parameters must be known before an estimate can be made of the actual amount of smoke that a material will produce.

If the mass optical density of a material is a measure of the quantity of its smoke, the quality of smoke is determined by its toxicity. Smoke from virtually any common material obviously can have lethal effects, containing as it does carbon monoxide and other toxic components. In addition, however, the smoke may be irritating to the eyes and respiratory tract, so that those exposed are hampered from escaping by the fire, even when the smoke concentration is at sublethal levels. This "incapacitating" effect of smoke is probably very important in determining whether people can actually escape from fires, but is not something which is readily measured. No good tests for incapacitation now exist; thus the relative toxicity of smoke is usually given by its LC 50, or by the lethal smoke dose, the L(Ct) 50, which is the concentration-time product required to be lethal. Several methods now exist to measure the exposure of laboratory animals, usually mice or rats, to the smoke and to determine the amount of material required to produce death in those animals in a given period of time, usually 30 minutes.

Smoke toxicity has recently become a topic of much public interest, partly because of heightened consciousness about fire hazard and partly because of the wholesale advent of synthetic materials in our daily lives. Most commonly found combustible materials before the synthetic age were derived, directly or indirectly, from wood or other cellulose products. Although wood burns to produce dozens of combustion products, it nevertheless contains only carbon, hydrogen, and oxygen, so that the spectrum of combustion products likely to be encountered is correspondingly limited. Modern synthetics contain a number of other elements, including halogens, sulfur, and nitrogen, all of which give rise to pyrolysis or combustion products different from those associated with the celulosics. Nitrogen is also present in naturally derived proteinaceous fuels such as wool. It was largely the recognition that the scope of combustion products had expanded tremendously that prompted investigations into smoke toxicity.

Measurement of smoke toxicity

Measuring smoke toxicity requires that the material be pyrolyzed or burned in the course of the test method.[4,5] How this is done can greatly affect the toxicity of the smoke, so that different test methods give somewhat different results. When a material burns in a real fire, it usually does so under a continuum of thermal and ventilation conditions, so that its combustion products in such a fire are not necessarily well predicted by using a single set of combustion conditions such as those used in a laboratory test method. These difficulties have made the interpretation of smoke toxicity data somewhat difficult, and for this reason small differences in the smoke toxicity of materials are often not thought to be significant. Even where relatively large differences are noted between the toxicity of various materials, the burning behavior of the materials must also be taken into account before a judgment of actual toxic hazard can be made.

Burning behavior of materials

The intensity at which the material burns is determined by how readily it will produce volatile fuel vapors when heated. It is possible to plot the heat release rate, or more directly, the mass loss rate, of a material as a function of the amount of heat applied to a given amount of surface—termed the heat flux. Some materials exhibit a very steep slope in such plots; others are relatively flat slopes. Therefore it should be clear that a flammability test method that exposes a material only to a low heat flux does not give a good indication of how the material behaves at high heat flux. This is particularly important because real fires generally expose the material to sizable heat fluxes, especially in the latter stages of the fire, so that in small laboratory-scaled measures the flammability results often do not provide the kind of data necessary to predict how a material will behave in a real fire.

One practical consequence is that the results of treating a material with a fire retardant and evaluating the effects of the treatment with the use of low-intensity fire exposure may differ dramatically from the performance of the material in an actual fire. It often happens that the effects of the retardant are no longer evident at higher heat loads, so that materials that are made "ignition resistant" by fire retardants often burn vigorously once the material has been ignited.

These effects are usually most pronounced in thermoplastic materials, i.e., those that melt before they burn and that do not form a rigid char structure on burning. Materials that char or leave a sizable residue on burning are often less sensitive to changes in heat flux or have a burning rate that declines with time as the char structure on the surface of the material builds up. The simplest example of the latter is wood, a chunk of which initially burns quite vigorously but leaves a sizable fraction of its combustible material as a charred residue; further burning is by means of glowing or smoldering combustion, which takes place more slowly than the initial flaming phase. If the wood is thick, burning will slow down as the char layer increases and the volatile materials necessary for flaming combustion must diffuse farther and farther from the interior of the wood before they can be burned. Some fire retardants enhance a material's ability to char, and these are often more effective at elevated heat loads than are those fire retardants that only are effective after the fuel vapor has reached the flame. These latter, which operate as flame poisons, or scavengers of the reactive flame intermediates, are the most easily overpowered by increased heat loads, which supply the fuel vapor to the flame at increased rates.

Assessment of fire hazard

In the foregoing sections the dynamics of fire, the aspects of hazard, and the properties of materials that impact the overall threat of fire have been discussed. In this section, the actual buildup of a fire in a room and its associated compartments will be examined to try to determine how these factors all interact in causing human injury.

The most common scenario for fire deaths is the ignition of a mattress or piece of upholstered furniture by a cigarette. This scenario is about five times more important in fire deaths than any other single kind of fire. Such a fire generally begins in the smoldering stage and may smolder for as much as an hour or two. Rarely will burning continue indefinitely in the smoldering mode; transition to flaming combustion is generally the rule. At this point, the scenario becomes identical with one in which the furniture began flaming originally, most commonly by ignition from another source such as a burning wastebasket or from a heating or cooking appliance. In any event, the *circumstances* of the flaming combustion of a burning item of furniture or mattress are of particular concern in life safety. If the item is located in a medium-sized living space, perhaps 700 square feet, very little time is required after flaming combustion occurs before the conditions become untenable. Ignition of a 25-kg chair made of polyurethane and covered with a normal synthetic or natural fabric can produce a fire of approximately 1-MW intensity in 1 to 5 minutes. This time may be lengthened substantially, depending on the circumstances of ignition, but once the item begins burning vigorously, the development of the fire and onset of hazard are usually rapid.

As discussed in the earlier section, the hot smoke from the burning furniture collects in the upper part of the room, and, as burning continues, this hot layer increases in thickness and extends downward from the ceiling. Typically this layer will reach a level of about 3 feet from the floor after the item has been burning 1 to 3 minutes. Temperature of this hot layer depends on the size of the room, the intensity of the fire, and the thermal properties of the walls and ceilings. In general, however, it will be fairly hot, and very soon too hot to breathe. The temperature of the layer increases rapidly, so that it has reached approximately 392° F (200° C) within another minute or two after having descended. The reason this is important is that those exposed to the fire must escape through this layer. They may be able to crawl beneath it, but will nevertheless experience its heat and may be forced to breathe it. Therefore the time at which the hot upper layer descends to a point near the floor is usually the first aspect of hazard with which those exposed in the fire must contend. The concentration of smoke in the upper layer is still relatively low when it first descends to a point where it is likely to be breathed, and the heat is likely to be more immediately debilitating.

The situation is different if the same fire occurs in a larger space, perhaps several thousand square feet, or if those exposed are farther from the fire source, e.g., down the hall from an apartment containing the fire. In this case the walls and the large space involved are sufficient to absorb much of the heat generated by the fire, so that although the upper layer is sufficiently hot to be buoyant, it is no longer hot enough to be quickly lethal. In such cases the toxicity of the smoke can be expected to be more important simply because the heat hazard has been removed. Lethal or disabling conditions are more likely to occur in the small room because of temperature, and in the larger spaces because of smoke toxicity.

In reality, those exposed to this kind of a fire are usually within a few rooms of the fire, so that they may originally be exposed to substantial heat. However, once disabled, they may remain in the environment long enough to take on lethal levels of smoke, often determined after the fact by high levels of carboxyhemoglobin in the blood. This may be the reason fire victims typically show symptoms both of heat exposure and of smoke inhalation. Fires in large buildings receive a great deal of attention, although they do not account for a large fraction of fire deaths. For the reasons just stated, in such large buildings occupants may encounter the smoke after the heat has been removed and therefore are more likely to exhibit effects caused solely by the smoke.

The precise mathematic relationships between the burning properties of the fuel and the time available for escape are complex. In general, however, one's intuition is not a reliable quantitative guide to the hazard involved. For example, one might suppose that if it takes 3 minutes for smoke to fill 1000 square feet of living space, 15 minutes would be required to fill 5000 square feet. Owing to the accelerating rate of burn, only about 5 minutes is actually required. Similarly, if those exposed to the smoke in the former case will have received a lethal dose after 6 minutes, those in the larger space will have experienced the same dose after about 10 minutes, despite the fact that the smoke must fill 5 times the original volume. These facts underscore the premium to be placed on early detection of the fire and make apparent the benefits of owning and maintaining devices designed to warn occupants before hazardous fire conditions are reached.

FIRE FIGHTING AND RESCUE*

The six major factors to consider in the fire fighting–rescue process are listed below.
1. Building hazards
2. Response context
3. Fire dynamics
4. Personnel
5. Equipment
6. Occupant factors

Building hazards

Type of use. Different rescue procedures are activated for different types of occupancies; for an occupied dwelling or at a late hour, excessive rescue work may be required. If mercantile, the type of material contained therein is a critical factor, especially if any precautions or special equipment are required, e.g., foam units or hazardous material suits.

Other issues and concerns pertaining to fire fighting–rescue in a specific instance include consideration of the following matters:
1. Site location (Is it in close proximity to other vulnerable structures—such as multiple dwelling units, schools, hospitals, and nursing homes—that could involve special evacuation measures?)
2. Fire fighting and rescue operations (Is special equipment such as ladder trucks for quickly evacuating occupants, helicopters for high-rise rescue situations,

---

*Contributed by Lt. Walter P. Long.

and ambulances available at the scene for immediately treating and transporting the injured necessary?)

Type of construction. A building of first-class construction (steel and masonry) represents a less hazardous situation, particularly when the danger of fire spread is taken into consideration; more time can be devoted to rescuing occupants and to handling the material(s) that are present. If hazardous materials are involved, there is also the imminent danger of explosion with the emergence of toxic and flammable fumes.

A second-class building (constructed of masonry and wood) can quickly and substantially be involved in a fire. When wooden joists and beams are heavily fire damaged, masonry walls may readily collapse when the fire spreads.

Third-class buildings are totally made of wood and present an urgent containment problem in a fire situation. The vast majority of dwellings in the United States are of third-class construction. The increased jeopardy to the occupants is reflected in the fact that most fire deaths occur in buildings of this type.

Building height. Since the maximum height of aerial ladders presently available to fire departments is 110 feet—with most being 100 feet—the height of a building is critical in the success of rescue and fire fighting efforts: a 100-foot ladder may possibly reach the tenth story of a building. With electric power usually being the first casualty in a fire, elevator usage is not considered a viable option.

The fire fighting and rescue personnel are heavily taxed, and their abilities greatly limited, when they have to carry fire fighting and rescue equipment by stairs, particularly at a high-rise fire. For example: SCUBA gear weighs 32 pounds plus the weight of a spare bottle or tank; protective clothing—boots, coat, helmet, light—weighs at least 40 pounds. Accordingly, the average fire fighter may have an extra weight load of 72 to 75 pounds to carry plus fire fighting equipment such as axes, lengths of hose, nozzles, first aid equipment, inhalators, stairchairs, and stretchers. In addition, the weight of forcible entry tools (e.g., bars, plaster hooks) has to be taken into consideration.

An extraordinary effort is required to support and relieve the initial fire fighting and rescue personnel involved in high-rise fire situations. This extraordinary effort can be ameliorated if safety features, particularly smoke towers and sprinkler systems, have been included in the construction of the building.

Fire site accessibility. To evaluate with any certainty how many people from a fire site may require treatment, it is essential to assay the accessibility of the fire site. The following factors affect accessibility:

1. Congestion (e.g., parked cars; delivery trucks; railroad cars on sidings; building, street, or road excavations; and even the presence of authorized vehicles, particularly of police and news media) can make direct access difficult.
2. Bystander interference and the accompanying hazard of their injury is ever present.

3. Other access obstacles, especially in urbanized areas, such as downed telephone and power lines and poles, the possible inaccessibility of water/hydrant supply (i.e., may be located at the rear of a structure or on the side of a cliff or require traversing a steep incline) or inclement weather conditions can make it impossible for fire fighting apparatus to reach the fire scene.

Floor load. A primary consideration pertaining to any structure involved in a fire is the weight load of the floors, especially in an industrial/commercial use situation when, in addition to the fire equipment and the fire fighting personnel, a great deal of water has been applied to the floor.

The weight load of roofs must also be taken into account. Heavy air conditioning units, tanks for storage of fluids, large chimneys, and billboards and other types of signs on the roof may present serious problems.

Construction hazards. Vacant buildings—buildings under construction, buildings under demolition, and buildings that have been involved in fires—may be occupied by a number of homeless people. Stairways, walls, and floors of abandoned buildings may be weakened and subject to collapse.

Newly constructed buildings present the following unique problems to fire fighting: makeshift stairways and wooden ladders going from floor to floor, unprotected openings (i.e., airshafts, stairwells), and building materials and equipment stored on floors blocking access to some parts of the structure, as well as the street.

Response context

Time and day. On the average, commercial-industrial structures will be heavily populated during daylight hours, whereas night hours are the most dangerous for dwelling occupants, especially in the early morning when most are asleep.

During the week traffic congestion can impact on securing a timely response. Over the weekend or on a holiday, business establishments—primarily in the office domain—are usually not occupied; and in dwelling units the occupants are likely to be awake and alert, and a fire is therefore less likely to gain extensive headway before being discovered, thus giving occupants a better chance to escape.

Climatic conditions

Temperature. The severity of a fire is correlated with the temperature of the outside atmosphere. In the northern climates, the winter season presents serious obstacles in handling fire fighting–rescue operations such as congestion of parked cars embedded in snowbanks and blocked and frozen hydrants and fire fighting equipment. Insulated dwellings where windows have been covered with pieces of plastic to keep out cold will also keep in heat and smoke and prevent occupants from hearing outside alarms.

In lower-income homes without central air conditioning, fire will spread more quickly because of drafts from open windows. In air-conditioned structures, the deadly fumes/smoke are distributed rapidly and the possibility that occupants will hear outside alarms is minimized because the building is completely closed.

Hot summer days with a briskly blowing, dry wind will cause fire to escalate to a conflagration with a concomitant fire storm. On the other hand, high humidity keeps smoke down and confined and the result is that heat and smoke are not vented rapidly.

Storms. During a severe storm—rain, snow, or heavy winds—the fire department will be taxed to its fullest. Delays in responding to a specific alarm can be expected when fire and rescue teams are involved in several emergencies at the same time.

Severe storm conditions will also likely result in power and telephone lines being down and fire alarm systems not functioning. When wires are blown against a building, electrical shorting will likely ensue, thereby increasing the hazards already present in effecting rescue in a storm situation.

Fire dynamics

Understanding fire dynamics may seem irrelevant to the treatment of victims; but the increasing use of new materials and construction methods, together with an increased concern for prevention, requires a sound knowledge of fire principles. Similarly, to understand the acute and long-term effects of a smoke inhalation injury, it is necessary to have an understanding of the fire, a basis for interpreting toxicity tests and research data, and timely use of modern therapeutic regimens.

Type, duration, and progress of fire. If, before arrival of fire fighting equipment, the fire has advanced to such a degree that heavy appliances have to be activated on the building, flying firebrands are being emitted from the fire, and the fire extends over and onto other buildings, fire fighting and rescue can be difficult. The presence of chemicals and other hazardous material in the area can also cause delay or additional risk. Similarly, possible explosive or electrical dangers must be considered.

Of concern is the growing prevalence of radioactive materials within hospitals and laboratories, particularly industrial laboratories, which must be recognized and dealt with at the fire scene. Ideally, these areas should be clearly labeled and previously made known to the fire department.

Conditions of stairways and fire escapes. Stairways without adequate fire doors and construction can easily become giant chimneys. Ideally the stairwells should be constructed of noncombustible material with appropriate fire doors, separately powered positive pressure ventilation systems, and multilingual signs with emergency illumination.

On occasion, alternate procedures must be put into operation because a fire is already consuming a stairway or is overlapping a fire escape. It is important to identify other routes for rescue and escape.

Presence of smoke or heat alarms and systems. Alarms and detector systems provide occupants of any type of structure with an early enough alert for a safe evacuation. Conversely, structures that do not have any alarm system are subject to greater fire advancement before discovery and therefore increased opportunity for injury.

Presence of wet or dry sprinklers. A sprinkler system is also a great asset in preventing or slowing fire spread. Water damage from sprinkler system activation is minimal when compared with its efficacy in preventing or minimizing loss of life. From a cost-benefit analysis frame of reference, sprinklers will not necessarily prevent a single injury or fatality; nevertheless, multiple injuries and fatalities are rare when a sprinkler system is properly in place.

Illumination. Lighting may be completely absent because of power failure from the fire. Confusion can then prevail, with occupants desperately trying to find exits and to find and assist loved ones, including pets. This situation is exacerbated when the elderly and the physically handicapped are involved.

Personnel

Number and proficiency of fire or rescue personnel

Staffing. Today's problem of undermanning may take a toll on fire department efficiency. Engine companies that once had one officer and at least four men are now down to one officer and two men. A crew of three men may find it difficult to search, ventilate, and rescue in a dwelling of two to three stories. Multiple alarms may thus have to be sounded to get more help. If life safety is involved, a delay is inherent in this response.

The highest priority for any fire department is life safety. This means that if there are people trapped in a fire, engine companies that arrive at the scene first may have to disregard setting up hose lines and proceed immediately to rescue operations. As a result, the fire may gain great headway, thus presenting an increased threat to other occupants of the building, as well as to the fire fighting and rescue personnel.

Specialized training. Today's equipment in the fire fighting–rescue domain is highly specialized; thus training in a number and variety of vocational-technical areas, including but not limited to the following, is mandatory: plumbing, electricity, carpentry, material packaging and storage, identification and handling of hazardous materials, building construction, rigging, motor vehicles, and other transportation modes.

Weather conditions. Fire fighters soon become exhausted from taxing their abilities in extreme weather conditions. Extended exposure under these conditions exacts a high price in fire fighter capability; frostbite and hypothermia may occur in severe cold weather, and heat exhaustion in hot weather.

Familiarization with building. There is no substitute for the familiarization of fire personnel with a building before the fire. Frequent tours, copies of building plans and fire procedures, and the prompt arrival on the scene of knowledgeable employees in industrial or public buildings can do much to enhance rescue and prevent further injury.

Knowledge of location and numbers of occupants. It is extremely important to be aware of the number and location of occupants. Sign-in logs are useful in this regard as is the placement of a label on the window of those rooms containing children or handicapped. Frequently, lives are lost in searches that are either unnecessary or conducted in the wrong area.

Availability of public utility personnel. Gas and electric companies must respond on many occasions to a fire scene. Leaking gas requires an immediate response to prevent an explosion; tangled outside wires on poles constitute a major hazard to fire fighting personnel and bystanders. But by the time the utility employees arrive, the area may be inaccessible to their equipment because lines of hose and other fire fighting apparatus impede their entry.

Equipment

Amount and type of fire fighting and rescue equipment. The question to be addressed is: Is the city or town equipped with the appropriate type and amount of basic equipment such as engine and ladder companies, fire alarm and communication equipment, adequate water and fire hydrant systems, and heavy rescue equipment to handle fires in the area?

SCUBA equipment. The day of the fire fighter going into an involved fire without protective clothing and SCUBA apparatus should be over. Although the time on the SCUBA tank can be considerably less than the 30 minutes usually identified, more time than this may be required, particularly in an extensive and/or high-rise fire; and provision must be made for spare equipment.

Other specialized equipment. Other specialized equipment that may be required—that is considered standard/available equipment available today to fire fighters–rescuers—includes the following: foam unit for handling flammable liquids, aerial tower for mass removal of trapped occupants, heavy-hose engine companies carrying 4- to 5-inch supply lines needed at large-scale fires to get water to the front-line engine companies, heavy-appliance engine companies for large-scale heavy-duty streams, and rescue units equipped with special extrication equipment.

Occupant hazards

Number and location. It is imperative to secure the best information possible concerning the number of people occupying the building, the number that have reached safety, and the exact location of trapped victims in any fire incident. Most fire-rescue personnel have been needlessly put at risk either because of misinformation concerning occupants allegedly trapped in a building or by people who, understandably, want immediate help for themselves or someone dear to them and who attempt to reenter the fire structure and get trapped.

Special population groups. Physically disabled persons, the elderly, children, and pets can present unique issues in handling fire fighting–rescue operations. Given the prevalence of pets in American society, it is appropriate to request backup from organizations such as the Animal Rescue League.

Physical condition and behavior of occupants. The physical and mental conditions are obvious factors in the effectiveness of rescue operations. Inappropriate behavior under conditions of stress are common. Occupants are often found in unusual locations such as closets or under beds. Panic can hamper both the fire fighting and the prompt location and extrication of victims.

Language barriers. With the rapid influx of refugee or foreign language groups (many under special visa provision and some unofficial), the problems of communicating urgent lifesaving directions and securing requisite social/medical history for emergency treatment are paramount concerns. The distinct possibility of deliberate communication of misinformation should be considered, particularly with those whose entry and/or continued residence in the United States could be problematic. But it is important for fire fighting and rescue personnel, as well as others involved in the health care arena, to have translation service readily available. At least one member in each fire fighting–rescue team should be familiar with foreign language term equivalents that may be needed in an emergency in the district.

REFERENCES

1. Bataille, P, and Vann, BT: Mechanism of thermal degradation of polyvinyl chloride, J Appl Polymer Sci 17:1097, 1972.
2. Benjamin/Clarke Associates, Inc.: Fire deaths: causes and strategies for control, Lancaster, Penn, 1984, Technomic Publishing.
3. Boettner, EA, Ball, G, and Weiss, B: Analysis of the volatile combustion products of vinyl plastics, J Appl Polymer Sci 13:377, 1968.
4. Clarke, FB: Fire hazards of materials: an overview, J Appl Polymer Sci 13:42, 1968.
5. Clarke, FB: Toxicity of combustion products: current knowledge, Fire J 77:84, 94, 101, 108, 1983.
6. DeRis, J: Chemistry and physics of fire. In Fire protection handbook, ed 15, Boston, 1981, National Fire Protection Association.
7. Friedman, R: Quantification of threat from a rapidly growing fire in terms of relative material properties, Fire Mater 2:27, 1978.
8. Gaskill, JR: Smoke development in polymers during pyrolysis or combustion, J Fire Flamm 1:183, 1970.
9. Henson, JLH, and Hybart, FJ: The degradations of polyvinyl chloride. I. Hydrogen chloride evolved from solid samples and from solutions, J Appl Polymer Sci 16:1653, 1972.
10. Lyons, JW: Fire: Scientific American library, New York, 1985, Scientific American Books, Inc.
11. O'Mara, MM: High temperature pyrolysis of polyvinyl chloride: gas chromatographic-mass spectrometric analysis of the pyrolysis products from PVC resin and plastisols, J Appl Polymer Sci 18:1887, 1970.
12. Smith, EE: Fire hazard characteristics of duct material, ASHRAE J, July 1972, p. 29.
13. Tatem, PA, Gann, RG, and Carhart, HW: Pressurization with nitrogen as an extinguishment for fires in confined spaces, Combustion Sci Technol 7:213, 1973.

3 Prehospital Care

EMERGENCY EVALUATION AND TREATMENT

The emergency treatment of the thermally injured patient starts at the site of injury. To fully meet this responsibility to both victims and fire fighting–rescue personnel, the health care provider should have a working knowledge of the four phases of prehospital care: in-fire evaluation and treatment, extrication, on-site evaluation and treatment, and transportation.

In-fire

The extent of in-fire evaluation and treatment depends on the on-site circumstances, including the rescue resources available. Unless the fire or source of thermal

Table 3-1. Evaluation and treatment of in-fire circumstances

Circumstance	Evaluation	Treatment
Extreme danger	None	None
Limited danger	Primary survey	ADCD
No danger	Primary and secondary survey	Same as on-site*

*Limited by equipment.

injury is no longer present, it is unusual for the rescue personnel to be able to provide any evaluation or treatment before extrication from the fire scene to a secure on-site location. At times, however, it may be possible to provide a primary survey consisting of the "ABCDs" (airway, breathing, circulation, and dangerous bleeding, i.e., bleeding from a major accessible artery). In these cases the treatment is appropriate cardiopulmonary resuscitation and pressure on the bleeding vessel, together with careful attention to the possibility of spinal injury; any specific care of the burn wound need not be addressed in the on-scene rescue operation.

As shown in Table 3-1, when there is an immediate danger to either the victim or the rescuers, extrication is paramount. Although the risk of added injury by moving at this time is a distinct possibility—and given that treatment, or even evaluation, is difficult and dangerous at the scene of the fire—relocating the victim may be the only viable option for survival.

On the other hand, in some instances a full primary and secondary survey may be conducted safely, and some degree of appropriate treatment administered. This can occur when the fire has been extinguished, but more often when the thermal injury is caused by something other than flame. In this event, and if at all possible, the rapid application of water, to both extinguish smoldering clothing and to lessen the injury by cooling the burn wound, is paramount. The most expeditious means of accomplishing this is with the use of the fire hose, since rescuers are rarely able to carry sufficient water for this purpose.

But in all cases of in-fire evaluation and treatment, the following points apply:
1. The amount of equipment that the rescuer can carry is severely limited.
2. It is difficult to find a safe and adequate work space.
3. The victim must be rapidly packaged for extrication.

Extrication

Ideally, injured persons should be moved only when they are stable. Fire scene circumstances do not often permit this option; in many instances removal or extrication must be performed quickly. Removal, therefore, from the danger area is usually in any manner possible consistent with protection of the victim from further injury and the safety of the rescuer.

First, the decision must be made to treat or remove. It is difficult to carry enough equipment to treat in a fire situation, plus it creates a hazard to the rescuer and further exposure of the victim to additional injury. Even a primary survey is performed only if the condition or situation permits (e.g., burns from hot liquids, electric shock).

If, on a prima facie basis, the victim appears to be deceased, the obligation to extricate at this time will vary between jurisdictions. If there is any doubt whatsoever, the victim should be removed, and treatment provided as warranted. Many victims of smoke inhalation and thermal injury may have stopped breathing but are still candidates for resuscitation. It should be emphasized that this determination cannot readily be made at the fire scene with the certainty required by law.

On-site

Primary survey. On-site refers to a safe position at the fire scene, preferably in a sheltered location, with good lighting such as in an ambulance, wherein primary (1 to 2 minutes) and secondary (3 to 4 minutes) surveys can be performed. Even if previously performed, these surveys should be repeated.

The generalized protocol for performing an on-site evaluation with concomitant treatment procedures is as follows:
A. Primary survey—life-threatening items
B. Treatment of immediate life-threatening items
C. Secondary survey
  1. Primary injury—thermal
    a. Percent TBSA, rule of nines
    b. Degree (first, second, third, or fourth)
    c. Location
    d. Smoke inhalation
  2. Other major injuries or diseases
  3. Past and social history
D. Treatment of nonlife-threatening conditions
E. Preparation to move

The items are listed in the order of priority and, as noted, include other aspects such as evaluating for other diseases and injuries, taking a social and medical history, treating nonimmediate life-threatening conditions, and transporting preparations.

Resuscitation. Immediate lifesaving care at the on-site level takes the form of cardiopulmonary and ventilatory support and precedes the care of the burn wound. Only the simplest and most readily available equipment—such as airways and Ambu bags—is required. This lifesaving equipment is considered more desirable than, for example, resuscitators that require a relatively high level of proficiency for their use and ongoing maintenance.

Secondary survey
Burn wound

RULE OF NINES. The rule of nines, the model for identifying the body surface area involved in a thermal injury, is presented in Fig. 3-1. This figure is usually reported as a percent of the total body surface area (TBSA) burned.

There are several advantages to this model: it is reasonably accurate, relatively easy to use, and readily remembered: head and neck, 9%; anterior and posterior trunk, 18% each; each upper extremity, 9%; each lower extremity, 18%; and the genitalia, 1%. This model is valid only for patients over the age of 4 years, but at this treatment level it will suffice.

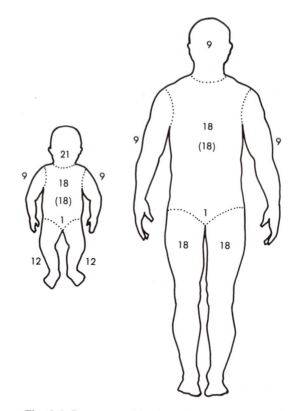

Fig. 3-1. Percent total body surface area (TBSA).

BURN DEPTH VS. CLINICAL FINDINGS. Accuracy in determining the degree of burn injury is not an essential factor at this stage. What is important is distinguishing between major and minor burns for effecting treatment deposition. In Table 3-2, the degree of burn (first, second, third, or fourth) is displayed relative to its clinical signs and symptoms. The term "fourth degree" is not used often, but it can be useful in very severe injuries.

An example of a third- and fourth-degree burn of the arm is seen in Fig. 3-2. The translucency of the third-degree area and the clearly visible coagulated blood in the superficial vessels are pathognomic of this degree of burn injury. The exposed elbow joint is typical of a fourth-degree injury.

Table 3-2. Signs and symptoms of burn degree

Degree	Signs	Symptoms
First	Erythema	Pain
Second	Erythema, blisters	Pain, shock
Third	Gray-brown	Shock
Fourth	Black or charred	Profound shock

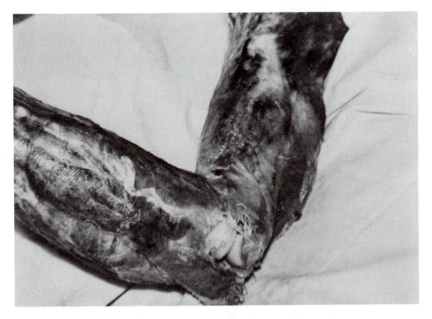

Fig. 3-2. Fourth-degree burn exposing elbow joint.

LOCATION. The location of the burn is not only important in assessing the total area involved, but often indicates the presence of other injuries (e.g., a facial burn is suggestive of an inhalation injury).

SMOKE INHALATION. The determination of the presence of a smoke inhalation injury at this juncture is important, primarily so that prompt cardiopulmonary resuscitation (CPR) and ventilatory support can be instituted.

OTHER MAJOR INJURIES OR DISEASES. Before transporting, it is necessary to assess the presence of other critical injuries or diseases. The most prevalent of these are as follows:

1. Trauma: penetrating wounds, blunt trauma, fractures, and spinal cord injuries
2. Diseases: cardiopulmonary, neurologic, or metabolic

Determination of these conditions can be made by using the standard techniques described in an emergency medical technician or paramedic handbook.

MEDICAL AND SOCIAL HISTORY. When a victim enters the health care system, the emergency room personnel are often faced with a major problem: minimal knowledge about the victim, with the rescuers being the only source of information. The primary concern is to identify the history of previous injuries and diseases, previous medication or drug use, and allergies.

Treatment of nonimmediate life-threatening conditions. At this point, only enough clothing should be removed to evaluate the patient. The patient should not be exposed to adverse elements. Clothing adherent to the burn wound and that which is necessary to protect the patient should be left in place.

Cold water. The prompt application of water, preferably cold, can be lifesaving and will also reduce the depth and extent of the injury. The application of water not only extinguishes the fire rapidly, but cools the tissue because of the obligatory heat of evaporation, thus minimizing the damage and reducing the pain. Thus the temperature of the water is not as important as its prompt application and its cooling effect when it evaporates. Later, when the situation is less emergent and for the first 24 hours, colder water or ice water controls the pain better. If sterile water and linens are immediately available, they should be used. In practice, the use of fresh water, i.e., water not stored for over 24 hours at room temperature, and clean rather than sterile linen results in almost no bacterial contamination. Similarly, the use of saline is not important during this short duration of treatment. The only contraindication to this treatment is abnormal chilling in cold weather.[6]

Topical agents. Over the years everything has been used. The best treatment at this stage is to use nothing except water and to protect the wound.

Smoke inhalation injuries. The treatment of smoke inhalation at the on-site location is nonspecific and consists only of CPR as necessary. A special caution is that, following an initial asymptomatic period, symptoms and signs often occur that require monitoring. Therefore, if there is any suspicion that this type of injury might have occurred, those exposed should be closely observed while awaiting transportation to a medical facility for further evaluation.

Fluid resuscitation. The following are guidelines for fluid resuscitation at the fire site:

1. Nothing by mouth because extent of thermal or other injury not known and all major burns develop ileus
2. Fluid or IV usually not necessary for short (i.e., less than 1 hour) period
3. If available, Ringer's lactate, at rate determined by formulas (see Chapters 7 and 9)
4. If long duration and IVs not available, then austere medical practice—as described in Chapter 13

As noted in the list, although IV fluids represent the optimum treatment, a delay of 10 to 15 minutes is usually not critical. If transportation will take longer, or if there has been a delay between injury and rescue, this delay could escalate the care situation to a critical level of concern.

To date, the value of the administration of IV fluid at the site has not been verified on a systematic clinical trial basis. However, with the widespread use of paramedic programs capable of on-site administration of IV fluids, this information will likely be verified in the near future.

TRANSPORTATION
Time factor

When to transport is a critical factor in resuscitating the victim. This decision has to take into account the capability and resources of the rescue team and that of the envisioned receiving facilities, including consideration of time-distance factors and the number and type of injuries/victims to be transported. The following is a summary of the factors involved in transporting thermal injury victims from an on-site location:

1. Safety to victim and rescuers
2. Condition of victim
3. Availability and mode of transportation
4. Duration of move
5. Availability of alternate destination
   a. Field care
   b. Emergicenter
   c. Local hospital
   d. Major hospital
   e. Trauma/burn center

Method

Manual vehicles. The manual method is severely limited by number and strength of personnel and distance. Many types of litters are available and can be used to further transport the patient to the hospital facility without unnecessary movement.

Land vehicles

Truck or car. In most vehicles the patient cannot lie down, nor is space available for providing resuscitation and other assistance. In wagons or trucks, exposure to weather elements is a factor and not recommended unless the patient is stabilized.

Ambulance. Ambulances are usually well equipped and, except for cosmopolitan ambulances, personnel have room to work. A trip of any distance is still not recommended until the patient is properly stabilized and packaged.

Air vehicles[5]

Helicopter. This means of transportation seems to have an element of mystique, and, indeed, its proper use can be lifesaving; but it must be remembered that it is almost impossible to care for the patient in flight because of noise, vibration, space, or exposure.

Fixed wing. Overall, fixed wing is better than helicopter if the aircraft is properly fitted and equipped and the patient has been cleared by someone knowledgeable in the adverse aspects of the physiology of flight such as lowered atmospheric pressure and partial pressure of oxygen. It is still difficult to work on the patient during transit, and adequate stabilization and packaging are mandatory before flight. With the exception of the U.S. Air Force C9 fleet, few aircraft are designed as aeromedical evacuation aircraft; all must compromise at some level.

Packaging

Packaging of the patient for transport includes the following:
1. Dressing or coverage of the wound
2. Support equipment and all other details (e.g., preparation of resuscitation apparatus and enroute supplies, protection of the burn wound with clean or sterile sheets and blankets, and splinting of major fractures and dressing of other wounds)
3. Necessary supplies and personnel for monitoring the patient
4. All medical records and detailed instructions to the personnel in the event of patient deterioration
5. Where and how to communicate to a base station.

Little thought of, but frequently needed, are specific directions as to destinations, since in many instances the transportation will be to an unfamiliar location.

Destination

Where to transport will depend on many factors referred to above, e.g., type of transportation, number of patients, distance to medical facilities. In general, "to the nearest facility" where resuscitation can most readily be started is the best rule to follow. Later the patient can be transported to specialized centers.

The following classification criteria are based on the recommendation of the American Burn Association and endorsed by the American College of Surgeons and by most state regulatory agencies.[1]

Classification of burn injuries[1,2,3,8]

Major burn injury. Major burn injury is classified as: second-degree burn of greater than 25% BSA in adults or 20% in children; any third-degree burn of 10% BSA or greater; any burn involving hands, face, eyes, ears, feet, or perineum; any inhalation injury, electrical burn; complicated burn injury involving fractures or other major trauma; and all poor-risk patients.

Moderate, uncomplicated burn injury. Moderate, uncomplicated burn injury is classified as: second-degree burn of 15% to 25% BSA in adults, 10% to 20% BSA in children; or less than 10% BSA third-degree burn that does not involve eyes, ears, face, hands, feet, or perineum.

Minor burn injury. Minor burn injury is classified as second-degree burn involving less than 15% BSA in adults, less than 10% BSA in children, and less than 2% BSA third-degree burn not involving previously mentioned critical areas.

There are a growing number of trauma centers in the country to which transfer might be desirable. Time and distance are always factors, and it is far better to transport to the nearest facility where resuscitation can begin or continue and the patient can be stabilized and evaluated. Thereafter, following communication with the trauma center, safe transport can be arranged.

There are now some 78 burn centers located throughout the country. At present these appear to provide sufficient beds yet only admit about 12,000 patients per year. Clearly, not all burn patients need to be treated in a burn center to receive optimum care. Similar to trauma center referrals, resuscitation is best started locally. The treatment program for the patient is then reviewed with burn center personnel and, if recommended, transferred to another facility.

Customarily all burn patients enter the health care system nearest the site of injury and thereafter are considered for transport to a hospital with optimal facilities such as a burn unit or trauma center, depending on distance and time, burn complications (i.e., respiratory distress or shock), and bed availability.

The importance of direct communication and transfer agreements is emphasized. If the seriousness of the injury dictates, the victim is transported to the closest qualified emergency department or special care hospital, possibly followed by a transfer to a hospital with optimum facilities that can be arranged after stabilization and initial resuscitation.

Although the destination following initial resuscitation will vary, depending on many factors, the prevailing guidelines reveal that patients with a major burn injury are best treated at a burn or trauma center. The patient with a moderate, uncomplicated burn can be treated at either a moderate or large primary hospital, depending on the expertise of the staff; a minor burn is customarily treated at a primary facility. In practice, usually because of location, burn and trauma centers often function as primary- and secondary-level providers in addition to their tertiary roles.

Communications

Good communication is essential if prompt and optimum care is to be given. Ideally the receiving medical facility should be included in the alert and warning network and should then be kept informed of the fire events. At least there should be as much notification time as possible before arrival, and the receiving facility should have the opportunity to assist by means of the emergency radio communications network.

Contact can be made to the dispatcher, hospital emergency room, or trauma or burn center. Usually radio is used for this purpose, and there should be a separate medical channel. The protocol to follow is given in the box below. These data are necessary to assist with on-site and enroute care and to prepare the emergency or receiving facility.

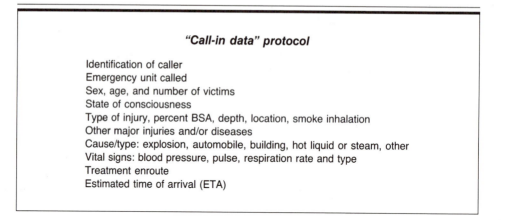

"Call-in data" protocol

Identification of caller
Emergency unit called
Sex, age, and number of victims
State of consciousness
Type of injury, percent BSA, depth, location, smoke inhalation
Other major injuries and/or diseases
Cause/type: explosion, automobile, building, hot liquid or steam, other
Vital signs: blood pressure, pulse, respiration rate and type
Treatment enroute
Estimated time of arrival (ETA)

Care enroute

At this point, because of the shock or the depth of the injury, victims are frequently not in pain. To sustain them and to treat any emergencies that may occur enroute require careful planning and training. Provision should be made to continue any cardiopulmonary resuscitation, and adequate supplies should be provided. The burn wound treatment with cool water should also continue, as well as that for other diseases or injuries. The psychologic aspect of care is very important during this period. Patients need reassurance concerning their own survival and that of other family members.

RECORD-KEEPING

In addition to the requirement to maintain accurate records upon which to base the continuing care of the patient, it is mandatory to preserve the legal rights of the patient in the event of any future liability. Furthermore, given the pervasive nature of personal liability suits in American society, proper record-keeping is the best insurance possible. Finally, it should be emphasized that many of the presently effective new methods of prevention and treatment are based on the analysis of the data secured from these types of records.

For the maintenance of a quality assurance program throughout the emergency medical care system, records are absolutely indispensable for analyzing mortality and morbidity trends and for securing an empirical foundation for future programs.

In summary, the following data sets should be kept in the forefront when considering which records pertaining to the thermal injury are needed:

1. Fire injury incident data
2. Medical and social history
3. Treatment and progress data

INTERHOSPITAL TRANSFERS

Interhospital transfers are discussed at this time because of the frequent consideration to bypass local facilities in favor of those more distant but better equipped. Almost without exception, transfer to the nearest facility offering basic resuscitation is preferable to incurring distance and delay. Thereafter interhospital transfer should be considered consistent with prior policies and procedures that result in agreements noted as "compacts." These compacts can then be used to determine when, how, and if the patient is to be transferred. The general guidelines that are consistent with today's practice concerning interhospital transfers are discussed in the following paragraphs.[7]

Indication

Sound rationale for an interhospital transfer is that the referring hospital does not have the capacity, resources, or special technical expertise to care for the patient. But in a study by Schiff and associates[7] in 1986, it was reported that, of 467 patients transferred, 24% were in an unstable condition with concomitant increase above the expected mortality. It was their conclusion that the transfers were predominantly for economic reasons. Unfortunately, under the present diagnosis-related group (DRG) and other cost saving programs, this tendency will likely persist, with the distinct possibility of an increase in transfers.

Timing

If at all possible, all patients should be stabilized before transfer. In any case, resuscitation, particularly respiratory and fluid therapy, should be well in progress.

Location

Where to transfer will depend not only on the severity and type of patient injuries, but also on the distance and capability of the receiving facility. Transfer protocols and arrangements should be part of every hospital's policies and procedure guidebook and should be approved by both facilities before the need arises.

Communication should be direct between the treating physicians and, particularly with burn patients, between physician and nursing staff. Medical records should be complete, with follow-up provision for forwarding the results of any laboratory tests in progress.

Method

Although there are many methods of transport, each has the same limitations described previously. And, unlike the initial transfer, the patient will benefit more from further stabilization than if he is transported by means of an inadequate method that causes further injury or delays proper treatment.

REFERENCES

1. American Burn Association (ABA): Specific optimal criteria for hospital resources for care of patients with burn injury, Dallas, 1976, American Burn Association.
2. Baker, SP, et al: The injury severity score: a method for describing patients with multiple injuries and evaluating emergency care, J Trauma 14:187, 1974.
3. Cayten, CE, and Evans, W: Severity indices and their implications for emergency medical services research and evaluation, J Trauma 19:98, 1979.
4. Edlich, RF, et al: Firefighter's guide to emergency rescue and care of victims burned in structural fire, J Burn Care 4:367, 1983.
5. Harvey, JS, Cruse, CW, and Sherman, RT: Aeromedical evacuation: a method for transporting critically ill patients, J Burn Care 3:377, 1982.
6. King, TC, Zimmerman, JM, and Price, PB: Effect of immediate short-term cooling on extensive burns, Surg Forum 13:487, 1962.
7. Schiff, RL, et al: Transfers to a public hospital: a prospective study of 467 patients, N Engl J Med 314:552, 1986.
8. Tobiasen, J, Hiebert, JM, and Edlich, RF: A practical severity index, J Burn Care 3:229, 1982.

4 Emergency Room Assessment

OBJECTIVE AND SCOPE

Emergency room assessment is a continuous, dynamic process coupled with care of the patient. However, there are steps into which the assessment, review, and planning processes can be logically divided.

Primary survey

A rapid preliminary evaluation or primary survey is extremely useful at this point. This can be performed concomitantly with resuscitation efforts and should provide an adequate basis for treatment until resuscitation and stabilization procedures are well under way, often a period of 1 to 2 hours. At that time a full conference review and assessment follow.

The assessment format, including treatment priorities, for a patient with major thermal injuries follows.

1. a. Determine need for any immediate lifesaving measures (e.g., CPR)
   b. Treat immediately
2. Determine if major or minor thermal injury
3. a. Evaluate for other major injuries or illnesses
   b. Start resuscitation (i.e., insert IV needles, draw blood for laboratory and determination of ABGs, start Ringer's lactate, insert Foley catheter)
4. Make preliminary evaluation
5. Complete history, physical and radiologic examinations, laboratory tests, photographs
6. Review in detail and analyze laboratory results
7. Analyze clinical monitoring
8. Readjust clinical program
9. Assess special problems

Although there can be some question whether the patient has a major injury, this procedure should be used unless there is a definitive evaluation indicating otherwise. It is not uncommon to discover that a victim's major problem may not be the result of the thermal injury, but initial case evaluation and resuscitation procedures are usually identical for any major problem.

Type of thermal injury

There is a time immediately following the primary survey and the initiation of any required lifesaving measures to determine whether the thermal injury is of major or minor consequence. The determination at this point is made on the basis of the results of the primary survey, i.e., the need for immediate CPR, which would obviously place the injury in the major category, a rapid assessment of the vital signs, the approximate percent of BSA involved regardless of the depth, the location of the injury, and the presence or absence of other injuries or illnesses.

Other serious injuries or illnesses are often overlooked in the charged atmosphere surrounding a burn patient. Among the most serious are myocardial infarctions, fractures of the pelvis or femur, blunt trauma injuries of the abdominal organs, metabolic abnormalities, and chemical intoxication.

Cardiopulmonary resuscitation

In the primary survey it is always necessary to assess the requirement for an immediate lifesaving procedure such as CPR in the form of airway placement, ventilatory support, external cardiac massage, and stopping of major accessible bleeding. The immediate requirements to proceed to IV fluid and medication therapy and possible relief of hemothorax and pneumothorax are not unique to the burn patient but prevail for all patients entering an emergency treatment facility.

Secondary survey

Fire and health history

Fire data. Although fire data may not seem important at this stage in the resuscitation of a major burn, the data are often irretrievable later when this type of information could help explain therapeutic enigmas, aid in prevention, and be of importance in any possible liability follow-up that could ensue. Essentially, what is needed is whether the incident correlates with the injury. Are there any unusual circumstances? In this regard, the following questions related to the fire are critical:

1. Where was it?
2. In what type of building or surroundings did it occur, and how was it used (i.e., warehousing, manufacturing, products involved)?
3. How did the fire start and in what sequence?
4. Where was the victim found?
5. Under what circumstances and how was the rescue effected?
6. What was the environment surrounding the patient at the time?
7. Were there drugs, alcohol, or any medications nearby?
8. What did the fire fighters or rescue personnel learn from the family or patient that related to the circumstances involved or the prior medical history of the victim?
9. What treatment, particularly respiratory support, had the patient received following rescue, and for how long a duration?
10. Is there any history of a closed-space exposure?

Health history. A complete and extensive history at this time often seems irrelevant; yet the need rapidly becomes evident when an attempt is made to manage the postburn events. Obtaining the history is a continuing process, necessitating periodic reviews and weighing of the import of new data. For a comprehensive history, all systems should be included, with emphasis not only on the present events, but on history of past illnesses and injuries, medication, allergies, and psychiatric and social circumstances.

Evaluation of shock status

Blood pressure and pulse. It can be difficult to obtain blood pressure and pulse rate in a severely burned patient because of burns of the extremities and subsequent edema, hypotension, and vasoconstriction. The presence of the cuff may continue to macerate the burn wound.

If treatment is to be implemented, it is mandatory to obtain a pressure both for evaluation and monitoring, although use of the blood pressure and the pulse rate only correlates moderately with perfusion of vital organs and cannot be directly used for treatment purposes.

It is also not uncommon for a severely burned patient with involvement over 90% of the BSA to have no obtainable blood pressure, but be pain free and conscious for as long as 12 to 24 hours before coma and death ensue.

Temperature. Core temperatures such as rectal or esophageal are the only reliable sources. The temperature is usually subnormal as a result of continued insensible water loss with its obligatory energy requirement, and aggravated by treatment with topical cold water applications. In fact, this is so much the rule that any elevation should make one highly suspicious of a septic process.

It should be noted that hypothermia is more common in gram-negative sepsis than is a febrile reaction. High fever occurring within the first day or two postburn is more often associated with either atelectasis or a streptococcal infection, and on the basis of clinical findings, even without laboratory confirmation, should be so treated, often as a therapeutic test.

Respiration. Observation of the rate and type of respiration can provide an early diagnosis of obstruction or other forms of respiratory distress. Recording of these data is also an excellent method of monitoring the resuscitation efforts.

Renal and pulmonary functions. If adequate urine output reflects adequate perfusion of the kidneys and the other vital organs, the urine output can be used both as an assessment of the degree of shock and as a means of monitoring the resuscitation. This correlation is true in the majority of cases and can be presumed so until proven otherwise.

Every major thermal injury, including those with relatively minor burns but associated either with smoke inhalation or concomitant cardiopulmonary disease, requires an indwelling urinary catheter to be placed and timely measurements. Parameters to be monitored include output and rate, specific gravity, and presence of hemoglobinuria or glycosuria.

The use of central venous pressure, pulmonary wedge pressure, and Swan-Ganz lines is discussed further in other sections.

Physical examination. The physical examination should include the standard areas of concern: present illness/injury; past history, including medications and allergies; and a system review. A thorough physical examination should also be performed, including eye, breasts, pelvic, rectal, and other areas often overlooked in the acute situation when the principal diagnosis appears evident.

BURN WOUND

The patient should be examined completely for both the extent and depth of burn. Often this cannot be thoroughly performed without interrupting the resuscitation efforts. When the patient is stabilized and placed on a wash table or similar apparatus, a burn chart should be completed using the rule of nines or preferably a Lund-Browder chart (Table 4-1), which also details depth and age differences. It is not unusual to need to correct prior highly erroneous estimates.[4,6]

The determination of depth at this point is often difficult, since the systemic effect, i.e., the hypovolemic shock, is similar in both the second- and third-degree

Table 4-1. Lund-Browder chart: percent BSA according to age

Part of body	0-1 years (%)	1-4 years (%)	5-9 years (%)	10-15 years (%)	Adult (%)
Head	19	17	13	10	7
Neck	2	2	2	2	2
Anterior trunk	13	17	13	13	13
Posterior trunk	13	13	13	13	13
Right buttock	2.5	2.5	2.5	2.5	2.5
Left buttock	2.5	2.5	2.5	2.5	2.5
Genitalia	1	1	1	1	1
Right upper arm	4	4	4	4	4
Left upper arm	4	4	4	4	4
Right lower arm	3	3	3	3	3
Left lower arm	3	3	3	3	3
Right hand	2.5	2.5	2.5	2.5	2.5
Left hand	2.5	2.5	2.5	2.5	2.5
Right thigh	5.5	6.5	8.5	8.5	9.5
Left thigh	5.5	6.5	8.5	8.5	9.5
Right leg	5	5	5.5	6	7
Left leg	5	5	5.5	6	7
Right foot	3.5	3.5	3.5	3.5	3.5
Left foot	3.5	3.5	3.5	3.5	3.5

Modified from Lund, CC, and Browder, NC: Surg Gynecol Obstet 79:352, 1944.

wound; but some attempt should be made to describe it. This difficulty in determining depth of the burn does not usually affect treatment.[2,3]

The difference in the BSA of adults and children should be noted (see Table 4-1). This difference is primarily seen in the head, which represents 9% BSA of an adult and 17% BSA of a 1-year-old.

Fig. 4-1 is a nomogram for both adults and children. Using this figure, it is possible to convert weight and height to square meters of surface area.

To determine the area of the burn in square centimeters or meters, the square meters of the patient's BSA are multiplied by the percent of the BSA burned, as determined using either the rule of nines or the Lund-Browder Chart. This method can also be used to determine the square centimeters of area grafted.

Although these data are not very helpful in treating the burn patient, they are frequently requested by health insurance carriers and therefore can be considered a necessary recording task.

To use the chart, a ruler is placed at the appropriate height and weight level, and the total surface area is read at the point at which the ruler crosses the square area, *S.A.* The same procedure is used for the determination of the burn area in children.

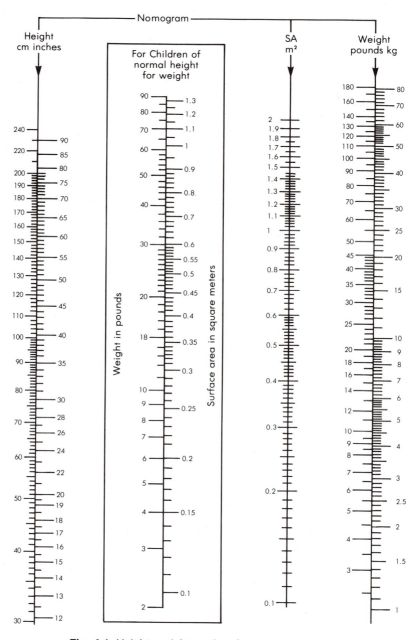

Fig. 4-1. Height, weight, and surface area nomogram.

INHALATION INJURY
Signs and symptoms

Early physical signs include the following: (1) the development of rales and inspiratory stridor caused by upper airway obstruction or bronchospasm, and (2) expiratory stridor indicative of upper airway obstruction and severe bronchospasm caused by edema and inhalation of an irritant or the inhalation of substances to which the patient is allergic. Both findings, particularly expiratory stridor, demand immediate treatment. Early onset of hoarseness and vocal cord lesions may be the result of nonspecific irritants or acid particulate matter. The findings of stupor or unconsciousness, facial burns, singed nasal vibrissae, bronchorrea, and sooty sputum are also pathognomonic.

Pulmonary assessment

Pulmonary complications are the major factor in fire deaths following admission to health care facilities and undoubtedly a primary contributor in causing in-fire deaths, although available data require more substantiation. In a recent study of those burn victims dying following admission to a hospital, smoke inhalation to some degree was a major factor in 76% of the deaths. But pulmonary complications do not necessarily mean that a smoke inhalation injury was the major contributing factor per se; the effects on the pulmonary bacterial host defense mechanism as a result of a major cutaneous burn can be devastating. What has happened is that patients still die of shock from massive burns and these are the ones treated and reported by the burn centers, which reporting can confound the analysis. Although burn wound sepsis is no longer the major cause of burn death, wound sepsis, and more important, pulmonary sepsis can be deadly.

Arterial blood gas (ABG) determination

No one test has more diagnostic value than the determination of arterial blood pH and gases. Ventilation and perfusion abnormalities (i.e., blood gas values and xenon-133 lung scan studies) can precede clinically apparent hypoxemia. Generally, a PaO_2 of less than 75 torr is diagnostic; there is also a marked metabolic acidosis in at least half the cases.

As a result of recent advances in equipment development, there are few hospitals that cannot readily and accurately make this determination. Some confusion may exist as to whether the sample is arterial, or it may be difficult to perform the arterial puncture in a severely burned patient, particularly in shock; but this can usually be accomplished from the femoral artery even at the risk of transcending burn tissue and before considerable edema has developed. Once the diagnosis has been made or confirmed and it appears that repeat or frequent determinations will either be required or difficult, a catheter can be placed in a convenient artery, preferably the radial; but even the femoral artery should not be ruled out in a risk/benefit evaluation.

Although it may appear that the simple identification of abnormalities in pH or blood gas values may establish the diagnosis, there are a number of pitfalls: the determination may be made too early following exposure; abnormalities may be caused by obstruction of the airway; there may be metabolic disturbances related to shock; the patient may have other nonassociated cardiopulmonary diseases related to, or independent of, the present injury; or there may be late-term toxicologic effects as a result of inhalation of a product of combustion. Despite these pitfalls and since treatment is usually nonspecific and proper treatment is directly related to the maintenance of normal pH and blood gas levels, these tests are critical.

Hypoxemia, significant if present, may initially be absent in 80% of patients who subsequently develop evidence of inhalation damage. Pulmonary dysfunction is noted in an increase in alveolar-arterial Po_2 gradient and a decrease in compliance.

Pulmonary function tests

There are a variety of pulmonary function tests that are generally nonspecific and related more to the irritant properties of a given pyrolysate and its subsequent edema formation. Although they may be of benefit in long-term assessment and care, they offer little more information than a basic history, physical examination, and continued monitoring of the patient (including determination of blood gases) provide. It should be noted that, in evaluating most inhalation exposure victims, baseline data are usually not available. Also of concern is the impact of a thoracic cage burn with the subsequent development of edema and decreased compliance. Pulmonary resistance tests can be as high as four times normal and compliance can be reduced by more than 50%. If smoke inhalation is suspected, the most valuable pulmonary function tests can be the repeat ones, either following initial observation or treatment.

Radiologic examination

The indications and findings of both chest x-ray film and xenon-133 diffusion studies are covered in Chapter 9.

As noted previously, routine admission chest x-ray films are mandatory to check for long-line positions, possible pneumothorax following long-line insertion, development of atelectasis, cardiac failure, sepsis, and presence or absence of associated cardiopulmonary disease. These procedures are safe and do not require patient cooperation per se.

If an inhalation injury is suspected, it is important to obtain the xenon-133 scan in the immediate postburn period. Usually this is best accomplished following initial resuscitation and stabilization.

Fiberoptic bronchoscopy

Fiberoptic bronchoscopy is a simple test that can be readily performed within the emergency room setting with about 90% accuracy. The primary findings are erythema, edema, and presence of carboneous material within the tracheobronchial tract. Further indications are a history of a closed-space fire, facial burns, and the presence of any major flame or steam burn.

ROUTINE TEST ORDERS

The typical routine test orders for those patients with a major thermal injury are as follows:

A. Hematology
   1. Complete blood count
   2. PT, PTT
B. Blood chemistry
   1. Standard chemistry profile with T4
   2. Serum electrolytes
   3. COHb*
   4. Ethanol and toxicity screen*
C. Renal function
   1. Urinalysis
D. Cardiopulmonary
   1. ECG
   2. ABGs
E. Radiology
   1. Chest x-ray film
   2. Xenon-133 lung scan*
F. Bacteriology culture†
   1. Wound
   2. Throat
   3. Urine
G. Other
   1. Photograph and chart wounds

Some are of immediate value, but most either provide overall background information about the patient or, most often, serve as a basis for further monitoring and treatment.

If the thermal injury has occurred shortly before admission, few of the laboratory results will affect the initial treatment. They will, however, be invaluable as a base-

---

*If indicated.
†Aerobic and anaerobic.

line for further resuscitation and to determine the preexisting health status of the individual or the existence of other nonthermal injuries or diseases.

Hematologic tests

Initial tests will show a moderate degree of leukocytosis. A failure of this response could indicate either an overwhelming gram-negative sepsis of an underlying, usually preexisting, defect in the patient's defense mechanism. In either case the finding is ominous, particularly during the first few days.

As a result of hypovolemia, especially during the immediate postburn period before the diuretic phase, there is a period of hemoconcentration, during which time the hematocrit may be as high as 55%. The tendency is to try to give sufficient fluid to dilute this figure to preclude the occurrence of renal shutdown and to prevent sludging of the blood flow through the smaller vessels. This tendency can easily result in precipitating an overload syndrome and is of doubtful value in preventing renal complications. In laboratory animals arterial flow has been shown to be improved with heparin or preferably low-molecular-weight dextran. Whether this is of value in patients is unknown because of the inability to sort out the effect of other factors. In any case, the dangers of attempted dilution surpass the possible advantages, as does administration of heparin. Small amounts, 250 ml/day, of low-molecular-weight dextran may or may not be of value, but are often given.

ABG determination

ABGs can provide some of the most useful information. Although the shock status is consistent with a lowered pH, the finding of respiratory acidosis will require adjustment of the ventilatory support, as well as the administration of sodium bicarbonate. Similarly, hypoxia may indicate an inhalation injury but could just as well suggest cardiopulmonary disease, which must be promptly treated.

Chemistry

Previously unrecognized or even undiagnosed disease entities are often detected during thermal injury testing. In the immediate postburn period there are few results that will affect resuscitation, but many will provide baseline data for addressing other problems.

Urinalysis

Using urine output for monitoring fluid therapy provides a means of recognizing diabetes or high output renal failure. Frequent determinations of specific gravity and glycosuria are most helpful in this regard. To fully manage the therapy, it is also important to determine urine electrolytes.

Special studies

Special studies refers to tests such as sputum cytology and specific tests for neurotoxic, hepatotoxic, and nephrotoxic effects. Extravascular lung water studies show an increase in vascular shunting and extravascular water in smoke inhalation injury, but these results are of little value in diagnosis, prognosis, or treatment. On the basis of present information, these tests are recommended only as part of a research protocol. However, it is strongly recommended that many toxicologic screening tests, including those for blood alcohol and legal and illegal drugs, be obtained, particularly in the patient who is in critical condition or in whom the diagnosis or management is not clear. Several days can elapse before results of these toxicity tests are available, and by this time, answers to treatment enigmas that have been encountered have often been found in therapy or simply overcome by events, thus rendering the tests more valuable in a forensic or research context than in clinical decision-making.

Wound cultures

Although the usual methods of obtaining and performing aerobic and anaerobic cultures may be useful (i.e., with a dry swab), unless the surface is moist and sterile, they do not reflect the actual events within the wound. Similarly, a culture of the exudate may only reflect surface and not invasive bacterial growth. These limitations can be overcome in several ways: preparation of the wound before culture; the use of a moist swab or saline wash; biopsy of the wound; and the application of agar plates directly to the wound.

Before taking a wound culture, it is important to prepare the wound by gently washing off the gross exudate. This method does not remove enough bacteria to adversely affect either the type or numbers of organisms cultured, but does reflect more accurately the status of the wound (i.e., the presence and extent of bacterial invasion). In addition, the use of a moist swab, together with the prompt inoculation of the plates or culture broths, may demonstrate sepsis in an otherwise sterile wound. Direct staining should also be considered for the possibility of a fungicidal infection.

Biopsy of the wound, coupled with a serial dilution culture technique, will give both qualitative and quantitative results. This reflects the possibility of invasive burn wound sepsis and also determines the degree. Biopsies should be taken using sterile technique and should be from 0.5 to 1 g in size. Because there are disadvantages in taking them (i.e., they may leave a full-thickness wound in an otherwise second-degree injury and the results only reflect the status of the wound in a limited area and must be extrapolated to assess the status of the remaining burn wound), they should be performed selectively and only when the information will influence the care. An example of when biopsy is valuable would be in a patient 3 to 4 days postburn if all other signs indicate that sepsis is not being fully prevented or adequately treated. Another common use is before grafting to better ascertain whether a graft will take. But the cost of taking biopsies is a major factor in determining their use. To overcome these drawbacks, another technique advocated by Lindberg and colleagues[5] is the use of blood agar plate in which has been embedded a piece of sterile gauze to use as handles. This plate is applied directly to the burn wound. With this technique, it is important to first cleanse the wound of all exudate and antimicrobial agents and to allow the plate to remain on the wound for at least 15 seconds before removal. An approximate colony count or, more significantly, a relative colony count, can then be made at 24 hours.

As with all these quantitative methods, subculture techniques can be used for qualitative bacteriology and antimicrobial sensitivity studies.

CHEMICAL INTOXICATION

Drugs are a difficult epidemic problem in the United States. Their effect can mask, confuse, and contribute to the problems of resuscitation. Fire, social, and medical history can all provide a clue and, together with the odor and physical findings, can create a high level of suspicion. Blood toxicologic screening tests should be routinely performed in all patients except those who obviously are not intoxicated. Serial tests are important, but an injection of Narcan, which can both make the diagnosis and treat the patient, can be given.

There are two major categories of drugs, the withdrawal from which can be a problem immediately postburn: opiates and central nervous system (CNS) depressants. Of these, most serious is the withdrawal from the CNS depressants, including alcohol, which can result in convulsions and cardiovascular collapse. Initially increases in heart rate and blood pressure with both types of withdrawal, together with gastrointestinal symptoms, can further confound not only the diagnosis but the treatment. It is also of concern that it often takes up to several days for the withdrawal symptoms to appear, depending on the drug, dosage, and individual variation. For example, withdrawal symptoms for a single drug can begin anytime from 2 to 7 days postburn.

The diagnosis of drug withdrawal symptoms in a major burn patient can be more difficult than usual because of the effects of both the injury and the treatment. A suspicion raised on the basis of history, physical examination, and response to treatment is very important. A feeling that therapy is not producing the expected results may be one of the first indications.

It is regrettable that the various clinical tests such as methadone and sodium pentobarbital trials, which can also be used to treat the patient and to assist in the weaning process, are of little value in a patient with a major burn injury.

Although it is important to eventually wean the patient off the drug dependency, during the immediate postburn period it is impractical. What is practical is recognition of the dependency in order to cope with the signs and symptoms and the provision of sufficient analgesia for pain control. As an aside, it is often a refractory response to analgesics that first indicates the presence of a drug dependency.

RELATED ILLNESSES AND INJURIES
Cardiopulmonary

It is common for cardiac disease to be adversely affected by the anxiety and stress of a fire situation, as well as by the inhalation of pyrolysates. In these instances acute myocardial infarcts are often overlooked because attention is directed toward the more dramatic events. Somewhat similarly, pulmonary disease such as chronic obstructive pulmonary disease and emphysema may also be unrecognized. Although the adverse effect may not be acute, the prolonged impact can be fatal, usually because of pneumonia.

Metabolic

Diabetes is increasingly common in the older population and greatly complicates resuscitation. In addition, under the stress of the burn injury, it has been reported that as many as 1% of patients with a major thermal injury develop a "pseudo" diabetes that is not present if survival ensues. The awareness of this occurrence can lead to its early recognition and treatment.

Trauma

Concomitant trauma is one of the major reasons for morbidity and mortality in patients who could have otherwise survived thermal injury.

Psychiatric

In a series of 67 patients,[6] over half of the patients admitted for burn treatment had preexisting physical and/or psychiatric conditions that increased susceptibility to injury. The following were reported: psychiatric factors, 35%; physical illness, 15%; social factors, 12%.

CHARTS AND PHOTOGRAPHS

Charts and photographs should be made of all burn wounds. In many states this is a requirement, but even if it is not, they are invaluable in record-keeping. The detailed written descriptions are time-consuming, usually inadequate, and often left to the member of the team least qualified to do the task. There are a number of readily available forms that use the Lund-Browder chart. They should be large enough to allow for detail; if the patient is a child, the child modification charts should be used. The wound should also be photographed from several angles and in color as part of the permanent record. However, neither the chart nor the photograph replaces a proper narrative description in the medical record.

In the immediate postburn period it is common to be unable to distinguish between a deep second-degree and a third-degree burn. Since their effect on the shock phase is similar, this should not be of great concern. It should be recognized that the variance between observers in determining the percent of total BSA burned can also be considerable, but within the perspective of the situation it rarely has any bearing on subsequent decisions.

However, there is always a word of caution to those who seldom treat burn injuries, and even for those who do so regularly. During the early phase it is routinely difficult to fully and accurately predict the extent and degree of burn and thus the subsequent events. This fact should be discussed with the patient and/or family.

PLANNING CONFERENCE

This is an extremely important step in providing optimum care. When the patient first arrives at the emergency facility, there is the immediate need to evaluate and perform lifesaving procedures, including CPR, insertion of IV lines, fluid resuscitation, and general assessment. There is then a period before formally addressing the burn wound itself other than by an approximate estimation, when all things can be put on hold for a few minutes while the records are updated and reviewed and an evaluation and treatment plan is formulated.

This plan should include participation by both senior and house staff, nursing service, respiratory therapist, and any appropriate consultants. Some of the major items to be considered are:
1. Review all subsequent test results and clinical monitoring
2. Review policy and procedure checklists
3. Readjust clinical program
4. Assess special problems
5. Attend to family, ethics, and social factors
6. Assign tasks
7. Prepare detailed treatment and monitoring plan
8. Review medical record for updating and completeness
9. Select time and location of next conference

The monitoring plan should be as specific as possible, even with the awareness that in major burn injuries change is constant and necessary. The identification of monitoring parameters and goals is paramount to success.

REFERENCES

1. Helmer, FT: Patient classification systems in burn care, Burn Care Rehabil 7:511, 1986.
2. Hinshaw, JR: Why burn severity is often misjudged, Arch Surg 83:459, 1961.
3. King, TC, and Price, PB: The early differentiation of full-thickness burns, Surg Forum 11:285, 1960.
4. Knays, GA, Crikelar, GF, and Cosman, B: The rule of nines: its history and accuracy, Plast Reconstr Surg 41:560, 1968.
5. Lund, CC, and Browder, NC: The estimation of areas of burns, Surg Gynecol Obstet 79:352, 1944.
6. Noyes, R, et al: Stressful life events and burn injuries, J Trauma 19:141, 1979.

5 Treatment

INITIAL TREATMENT
Priority of care

For the most part, emergency room treatment and evaluation continue on a parallel course. In the management of a major thermal injury, like that of other major injuries, a double matrix system is recommended with both a physician and nurse in charge, whose duties and scope of responsibilities have been discussed and accepted a priori.

Emergency room treatment has as its goal comfort or intervention directed toward possible survival.[17] The issue of whether or not to continue to treat is one that is best addressed after a professional evaluation and therapy that includes CPR and putting IV fluids in place.

The emergency room treatment categories are not equal in importance or in the amount of time in which they should be accomplished. The box on p. 58 lists the priority in which they should be addressed. First, as always, is CPR. In addition to external cardiac massage and ventilatory support, this includes clearance of the airway and insertion of a nasotracheal or endotracheal tube, respiratory support, correction of blood gas and acid/base abnormalities, and the use of whatever cardiac medication or procedure that may be indicated.

CPR is followed almost simultaneously by fluid management, including the insertion of long lines for fluid therapy and critical monitoring, as well as the early insertion of an indwelling urinary catheter. If immediate CPR and fluid management are obviously required, the detailed history and physical examination, including a careful appraisal of the burn wound, take a lower priority. Similarly, the care of the burn wound itself can often be more safely and better carried out following initial treatment for stabilization and detailed planning.

Immediate lifesaving procedures
CPR

Insertion of airway endotracheal or nasotracheal tube. All unconscious patients need an airway. A nasotracheal tube is preferable to an endotracheal tube for long-term placement. They are better tolerated, but may be difficult to insert. It is important to insert the tube early before edema of the oropharynx or of the neck makes placement difficult. A soft tube and intermittent cuff should be used if available.

Tracheostomy. A tracheostomy in a burn patient will always result in a severe, often lethal pneumonia as a result of the loss of the cough and physical mechanism whereby the respiratory tract rids itself of hostile material and the continued introduction into the body of microorganisms from the burn wound and the hospital environs. As such, it should never be done prophylactically. The only indication for a tracheostomy in burn patients is in those in whom a nasotracheal or orotracheal

---

Emergency room treatment categories and priorities

A. Immediate lifesaving
  1. CPR
    a. Insertion of airway or naso/endotracheal tube
    b. External cardiac massage
    c. Correction of acid/base imbalances
    d. Cardiogenic medication
  2. Ventilatory support
    a. Oxygen
    b. Assisted ventilation
  3. Relief of pneumothorax or hemothorax
  4. Arrest of major hemorrhage
B. Fluid management
  1. Insertion of access lines
    a. Peripheral vein
    b. Central venous lines
    c. Arterial line
  2. Fluid replacement
    a. Crystalloid
    b. Colloid

  3. Insertion of monitoring lines
    a. Central venous pressure (CVP)/Swan-Ganz
    b. Foley catheter
C. Burn wound care
  1. Pain management
    a. Cold water
    b. Analgesics
  2. Topical therapy
    a. Cleansing
    b. Debridement
    c. Antimicrobials
    d. Escharotomy
  3. Systemic
    a. Antimicrobials
    b. Other, i.e., steroids, low-molecular-weight dextran
D. Care of other illnesses or injuries
E. Psychiatric support
F. Prognosis

---

tube cannot be placed, usually because of extensive head and neck trauma with obstruction; but even in these cases, it should not be performed in the emergency room unless the facilities are especially designed and equipped for this procedure. There is no reason to do one after an endotracheal tube has been inserted on the basis that the patient will need one shortly or that the tube cannot stay in place for very long.[14]

Fig. 5-1 shows a patient with a third-degree burn and massive edema of the face 24 hours after injury. For prolonged use, the nasotracheal tube is preferable to an oropharyngeal tracheal tube, is more comfortable, and allows better oral hygiene. It is important to use a soft dual cuff that can be alternatively inflated, to take care not to injure the nares or the nasolabial fold, and to provide local care so the patient does not develop an acute sinusitis.

External cardiac massage. It is sometimes difficult to detect heart sounds due to a burn of the chest wall. There also may be some reticence to perform external compression because of possible contamination and further injury to the burn wound, but these are nonissues in this situation and standard cardiac arrest or ventricular fibrillation procedures should be promptly implemented.

Correction of acid/base imbalance. It can be presumed that acidosis exists in this situation, either because of the cardiac arrest alone or as a result of the hypovolemic shock and a diminished perfusion caused by the burn injury. The continued presence of acidosis will exacerbate the cause or adversely affect the myocardium and,

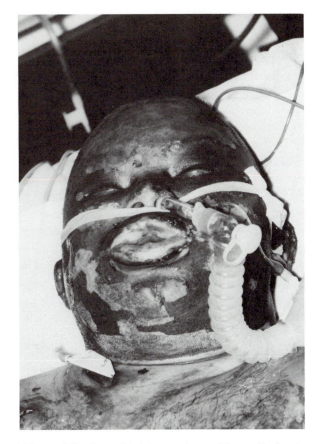

Fig. 5-1. Patient 24 hours following a third-degree burn of face with development of massive edema.

through shifting of the oxygen dissociation curve, degrade the already poor perfusion of vital organs. Thus it is important to address this condition. Usually the use of Ringer's lactate solution alone will be adequate to treat the acidosis caused by burn shock, but one should not hesitate to use intravenous sodium bicarbonate. One or two ampules may be given empirically as in any other cardiac arrest situation and thereafter as indicated by the results of pH and blood gas tests.

Cardiogenic medication. Specific recommendations for these classes of medication are not unique or contraindicated in the thermally injured patient.

Ventilatory support and treatment of smoke inhalation. All treatment is nonspecific, including respiratory support. Understanding the mechanisms will help in the treatment, planning, and prognosis. A clear airway with adequate ventilatory and respiratory support, together with serial determinations of arterial pH and blood gases, can be used to correct metabolic acidosis. Judicious fluid therapy is also critical and can be exceedingly difficult if there is some degree of cardiogenic shock.

Theoretically some inhaled pyrolysates have specific antidotes such as those for hydrogen cyanide. However, the rarity of the occurrence of these specific problems, the difficulty in their identification, and the inherent time delay on the basis of present knowledge precludes the use of any specific therapy for smoke inhalation with the exception of oxygen for carbon monoxide, which is also a part of nonspecific therapy.

Respiratory support. Chapter 7 discusses the use of various ventilators. Bronchodilators, oxygen, and corrections of acid/base imbalance are also common therapeutic modalities, but should be monitored closely. The need for a blood transfusion is rare and only indicated with preexisting disease or concomitant injury. Particularly since the use of an oropharyngeal or nasopharyngeal airway and the presence of bronchorrhea markedly alters the physical mechanism of the triad that comprises the pulmonary bacterial host defense mechanism and the second mechanism, the alveolar macrophage system may be diminished. Accordingly, it is obligatory that the tracheobronchial tract be kept as clean as possible. This requires frequent suction, often with lavage, and encouragement of the patient's own respiratory efforts.

OXYGEN. All patients with major thermal injury will benefit from some level of oxygen therapy. As a specific therapy such as for carbon monoxide intoxication, use of an endotracheal tube and 100% oxygen is mandatory. Giving oxygen to an emphysematous patient, which washes out carbon dioxide and results in apnea, is a nonissue in this serious situation; this problem can be identified later, and the patient appropriately weaned. Also a nonissue at this stage is oxygen toxicity, although it will be of interest and an important factor in the later development of atelectasis and sepsis resulting from the inactivation of alveolar surfactant and alveolar macrophage function.

ASSISTED VENTILATION. All patients with any indication of respiratory distress require an evaluation to assess the need for assisted ventilation. Controlled respiration is preferred to ventilate the patient more effectively and with less fatigue.

Relief of pneumothorax or hemothorax. Although pneumothorax or hemothorax is always a possibility as a result of other injuries, its presence is not uncommonly iatrogenic because of the attempted insertion of a subclavicular, supraclavicular, or inferior jugular vein access line. Although it is desirable to prove its presence with a portable or in-department chest x-ray film, physical examination can be most helpful. If the patient is having problems, at least a diagnostic needle thoracentesis can be readily performed. In the event of a pneumothorax, a tube with underwater seal or suction should be immediately instituted. Unfortunately, this may mean penetrating burn tissue, but that cannot be helped and should not be a deterrent, particularly in the high likelihood that the patient will require some type of positive pressure ventilatory support during the early postburn period as a result of external cardiac massage.

Arrest of major hemorrhage. Related injuries will occasionally result in major hemorrhage that must be addressed promptly. Bleeding can also occur secondary to treatment, such as after insertion of subclavian access lines or in escharotomies where the incision has been inappropriate or too deep. All of these instances may require appropriate transfusion, but they are generally unusual occurrences.

Fluid Management

Route. Time is important. Any route that can be rapidly used with even a scalp needle will permit time for the insertion of larger-bore needles or long lines such as subclavian or subclavicular lines. These lines can also be used for CVP monitoring and for fluid therapy if needed. Although there should be no hesitancy in the use of long lines, they really shouldn't be inserted until there is a full assessment and a plan whereby some veins are conserved for later use. If possible, fluid management lines should not be placed through burn tissue. When this is done, the infection rate and incidence of thrombophlebitis are considerably higher, and the insertion point also serves as a source of bacteremia.

Peripheral vein. The peripheral veins are often collapsed and subject to early phlebitis; thus it is difficult to infuse rapid, large quantities of required fluid. However, they can be accessed rapidly even through burn areas with a small needle to permit infusion of some fluid while the larger long lines are inserted.

Central venous lines. These lines can be placed either in the upper extremity through the jugular or subclavian vein or through a tributary of the saphenous vein. Ideally, they should not be placed through burn tissue nor should they be used for fluid replacement, medications, or laboratory tests. As a practical matter, they may have to be used for all of these, and the interpretation of their pressure values adjusted accordingly.

Arterial line. Arterial lines are useful, particularly if there is an anticipation of the need for frequent ABG determinations or blood pressure readings. In these cases, insertion, usually in the radial artery, should take place early, before edema makes it difficult, particularly if burn areas must be traversed in the process. If insertion through burned areas is necessary, the catheter is more likely to become infected and should be removed, cultured, and changed as often as feasible. Their use is acceptable in the overall risk-benefit analysis.

The placement of a right subclavian vein access line is shown in Fig. 5-2. In a critically burned patient with limited venous access, long lines are usually placed using either the jugular, subclavian, or femoral veins.

Occasionally the superficial saphenous vein can be used at the ankle. The advantage of this latter route is rapid insertion with minimal complications. Disadvantages are that it is not always available, it has limited size, and burn injury may be present. Table 5-1 summarizes the advantages and disadvantages of common venous access routes.

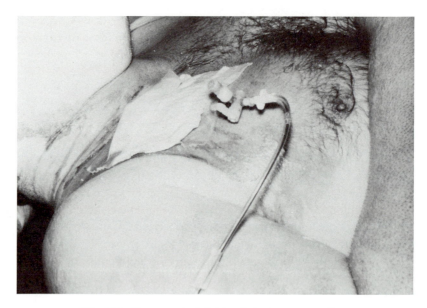

Fig. 5-2. Placement of right subclavian access line.

Table 5-1. Advantages and disadvantages of various venous access routes

Vein	Advantage	Disadvantage
Scalp	Readily available in infants	Very small
Hand	Readily available	Very small
Antecubital	Readily available Can use for CVP	Variable size
Internal jugular	Always present Large size Useful for all monitors	Requires time and experience Moderate incidence of pneumothorax
External jugular	Always present Large size Useful for most monitors	Requires time and experience Can be difficult to insert large monitors
Subclavian	Always present Large size Useful for most monitors	Requires some time and experience 5% to 20% incidence of pneumothorax
Superficial femoral	Always present Large size	Requires some time and experience
Saphenous	Usually present Medium size Few complications Basic experience only	Medium size Not used for monitors

Fluid replacement. Crystalloid refers to isotonic or hypertonic solutions, usually either normal saline, Ringer's lactate, or hypertonic saline solution. There are also varying concentrations of salt solutions commonly buffered and containing varying amounts of sodium, potassium, and chloride ions, and often varying concentrations of glucose, usually to enhance their isotonicity. These are discussed in Chapter 6. It is sufficient at this juncture to emphasize that the primary goal is to treat or prevent hypervolemic shock and to correct resultant acid/base imbalances. In treating a major burn injury at this point, issues of overload, possible cardiac failure, or caloric deficits are not of concern in comparison to the massive losses of fluid volume.

Time and volume replacement is more critical at this stage than the type of fluid infused. Ringer's lactate is readily available and functions effectively as a buffer. At this point in treatment, the sodium content is generally not a factor unless the patient is in obvious cardiac failure. But even these patients can be hypovolemic. The issue of colloid vs. crystalloid is never quite settled, but the administration of macromolecules or colloids has little or no effect on the hypoproteinemia or the reduction of edema through Starling's law.

Rate and amount. Although the rate can be adjusted later, it is important not to simply let large amounts pour in without accurate record-keeping and monitoring, should the fluid need to be more carefully adjusted following the initial assessment and implementation of an overall plan.

Insertion of monitoring lines. The use of CVP and Swan-Ganz lines to monitor the function of the right and left atria is also covered in Chapter 7. There should be no hesitance in the use of a CVP line, but the Swan-Ganz line does have some risks and is usually not needed.

Burn wound care

Analgesics

Indications. All conscious patients have pain and will benefit from analgesics. The severe pain usually lasts about 24 hours; subsequently medication can be reduced or limited to periods of cleansing and debridement or following physical therapy. Although addiction may be a problem in severely burned patients, it is not an issue at this time. However, the adjustment of suitable analgesic therapy in the addicted patient can be a problem. These cases need to be individualized.

Type. Meperidine and morphine are the most commonly used agents. Morphine has some sedative effect that may be helpful, and its adverse effect on respiration is usually outweighed by the benefits of pain relief and reduction of anxiety. Special attention should be paid toward determining the appropriate pediatric dosages.

Route. All analgesics should be given intravenously in order to ensure prompt action, controlled dosage, and predictable absorption. Small amounts given frequently are the rule. In practice, these drugs are best titrated to achieve maximum effect without oversedation.

Topical therapy

Immediate treatment. The immediate treatment is to cool the wound as CPR and the fluid management issues are being addressed. It is also important, as far as possible, to protect the wound from further injury or contamination. The wound can be cooled by the application of ice water, cool water, or room temperature water, since it is the obligatory heat of evaporation that cools both the wound and the temperature. Sterile solutions are desirable to reduce the number and type of bacterial contamination, but in practice nonsterile running water is acceptable during this phase for prompt cooling and cleansing.[13,26,37]

Debridement. Only tissue that is grossly necrotic should be debrided at this stage. Blisters serve to protect the wound from drying out from bacterial contamination. There is also less pain when the blisters are left intact. After a few days, the blister will usually break, and loose skin may be easily debrided during the daily wash sessions.

It is tempting to treat the burn wound by primary excision during the immediate postburn period. The problem with this procedure is the difficulty in accurately determining the exact depth of the burn and excessive blood loss. When excessive blood loss occurs during the shock phase, it can be disastrous. Excision, either full-thickness or, better, tangential excision, can be advantageous in deep second-degree and third-degree burns. In the past, before it was possible to control burn wound sepsis, excision had to be performed during this shock phase before the invasive burn wound sepsis could occur. Now it is possible to safely delay the procedure for as long as 5 to 7 days and still not excise through infected tissue. When this does occur, grafts slough, and bacteremia is common.

Because of blood loss, primary excision procedures are limited either to small burns or to use in children in whom massive and rapid blood replacement can more easily be accepted by the cardiovascular system.

The use of sutilains enzymes (Travase) has been advocated by some for debridement and preparation of the dermal bed for grafting within 24 hours. It has been most acceptable for use in deep dermal burns of the hands. Sterile sutilains ointment is applied directly to the burn wound. Degree of bleeding is used to indicate the activity of the enzyme and to confirm the clinical estimation of depth. The area is then covered with fine-mesh gauze impregnated with silver sulfadiazine (Silvadene) over which are placed heavy pads of normal saline. Although there is considerable pain, it can be controlled with morphine, and the dressings are changed every 4 to 8 hours until time of debridement. The debridement is carried out under anesthesia at 24 hours, using scraping rather than cutting action, and the area split-grafted.[44]

Tar and asphalt burns. Although tar and asphalt burns are not commonplace, they are not unusual among roofers and others whose occupation brings them in contact with such materials. Since tar adheres to the skin, the contact time is increased; the length of contact time, along with the high temperature, tends to produce much deeper burns than with other comparable hot liquid injuries.

Essentially it is most important to rapidly cool the burn wound and, in these cases, the burning agent. If this is started at the scene, so much the better, but it should be instituted or continued in the emergency room.

Removal of the tar is difficult and time-consuming and may cause further injury. It can be attempted following resuscitation and stabilization, or, if the burn is minor or time and resources permit, it can be attempted in the emergency room; otherwise it can be delayed until hospitalization.[20,38]

Petrolatum-based ointments are most effective for removal of the tar. Many antibiotic ointments are petrolatum based and also may be used for this purpose. Other agents such as polyoxyethylene-sorbitan may also be effective. It must be noted, however, that (1) these agents tend either to seal the wound or to further dissolve the lipids and further damage the tissue, and (2) the wound does not have to be scrubbed clean initially, particularly if complete removal would increase the morbidity or the mortality.

Topical agents. The principles governing the care of the burn wound are presented in Chapter 8. Although the quality of wound care is critical to survival, attention to quality can be safely delayed until the patient is fully evaluated, resuscitation started, and the patient stabilized.

Cleansing. Topical care starts with a thorough cleansing of the burn wound, i.e., irrigation with copious amounts of water before entering the hospital system, gentle washing with warm water using sterile gowns, gloves, caps, and masks, and a dilute detergent cleaner such as hibiclens or betadine. Ideally some spray mechanism is used for water debridement. This technique will serve to wash dirt, foreign matter, clothing, and loose skin from the wound. It will also reduce the bacterial count on the skin surface and, hopefully, eliminate some of the more virulent bacteria. Very important side benefits of this procedure are the opportunity, often the first, to closely and carefully examine all aspects of the wounds and the chance to chart and photograph them.

Antimicrobials

SYSTEMIC ANTIBIOTICS. No prophylactic antibiotics are recommended. Sputum cultures and gram stains should be obtained on admission and repeated daily as indicated. Antibiotics should be selected on a specific basis and with a plan for treating existing infections or those that may develop.

Those who advocate prophylactic systemic antibiotics specifically for streptococcal infections and those who believe that, should streptococcal infection occur during the first few days postburn, it can then be readily identified and treated are evenly divided. Even those who recommend prophylaxis limit the antibiotics to penicillin or its analogs, and the use of all others is reserved until a specific organism is identified. If there is any allergic history to penicillin, no systemic antibiosis is recommended.[15]

As with all other medications in this situation, systemic medication must be administered parenterally and preferably intravenously, to be effective. The recom-

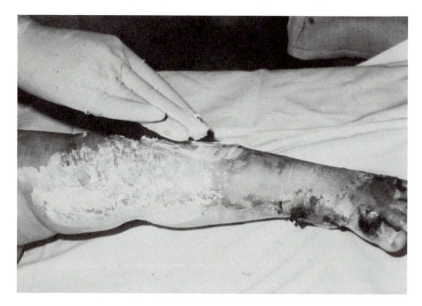

Fig. 5-3. Sterile glove used to gently cover wound with topical antimicrobial agent in cream base.

mended dosage for penicillin in adults is 1,000,000 U IV every 6 hours for 5 days or until the initial resuscitation is completed and specific cultures are available.

TOPICAL AGENTS. At present there are two topical agents commonly used to prevent and/or control burn wound sepsis. Silver sulfadiazine is a bactericidal agent that is basically surface acting. Sulfamylon is absorbed but is a bacteriostatic agent. Therefore, it is generally recommended that silver sulfadiazine be used initially unless the wound is already colonized. These two topical agents are applied twice daily following cleansing of the wound. Fig. 5-3 shows the technique of spreading topical agents about 0.2 to 0.4 cm thick using a gloved hand.

Immunization. Tetanus immunization is recommended for all patients with a major thermal injury, although it is difficult to find cases of tetanus reported in the burn literature. Standard recommended dosages are to be followed, but this medication can safely be delayed until the resuscitation process is under way.

At various times, immunization for other infections such as *Pseudomonas aeruginosa* and pneumococcal vaccines have been recommended. However, there is no clinical evidence at present that these therapies reduce either the mortality or morbidity.

Psychiatric support

It can be anticipated that all patients with a major thermal injury will require some level of psychiatric support to cope with their injuries and, most critical, any possible subsequent deformities and dysfunction. In addition, the patients' families will also require this type of assistance. The earlier the involvement, the better the result.

Prognosis

Much of the prognosis will depend on an unpredictable clinical course. This course can vary markedly. There are some general patterns, however. The first problem is airway obstruction, then pulmonary insufficiency, followed by a period lasting a few days of high pulmonary bacterial susceptibility. How these issues, including complications by the pulmonary effects of other injuries or diseases, can be dealt with clinically will largely influence the prognosis.

There is a most important correlation between inhalation injury and age or, even more important, between any cutaneous burn and the percent of total BSA involved in the injury, in which a dose-exposure curve simply shifts directly with age and with the presence or absence of other disease entities or injuries. The prognosis is also limited to the acute single exposure. No data are available as to long-term effects, although there must be some, particularly in those cases with extensive sloughing of the bronchial mucosa or the development of sepsis. They also occur, probably in the form of pulmonary fibrosis, as a result of stenosis at a tracheostomy site, or there is erosion of the bronchial tree due to long-term tube use.

Policies and procedures

An illustration of the initial treatment policies and procedures that should be addressed, discussed, and promulgated before the patient arrives is presented in the box on p. 68. These include issues that must be coordinated with both the nursing and administrative staff, as well as the various departments within the medical staff.

In addition, the box lists the various laboratory, radiologic, and special studies that should be routinely ordered for all patients with a major thermal injury.

Summary of initial care

Following a rapid preliminary assessment and resuscitation efforts, an overall review should be performed and the tasks and responsibilities for further evaluation, monitoring, and treatment clearly delineated.

CONTINUED CARE

Continued care is functionally defined as the care that is begun when the patient exhibits hemodynamic and ventilatory stability. It is the time when the emphasis is

---

Initial treatment policies and procedures

1. Notification of hospital staff of all patients with major burns either on admission or as soon as notification of transfer or transport is received
2. CPR started
   a. Airway established, avoiding tracheotomy and using nasotracheal intubation if possible and necessary
   b. Cardiorespiratory assist, if indicated
   c. Establish peripheral large-bore IV lines using Ringer's lactate
3. Evaluation of patient for other injuries and diseases
4. Treatment of high-priority injuries or diseases such as major bleeding, hemothorax-pneumothorax, major fractures
5. Insertion of Foley catheter: 16- or 18-gauge, two-way, with 5-cc balloon
6. Evaluation of burn
7. Treatment of burn with cool or ice water compresses
8. Immunization with tetanus toxoid if immunization greater than 5 years
9. If no immunization history, addition of Hypertet
10. History and physical record to include burn size and depth description, as well as associated complicating factors
11. Escharotomy, if necessary
12. Sterile technique: gloves, gowns, face masks, and hair stays
13. Lab work (record time drawn)
    a. CBC, diff, electrolytes, BUN, creatinine, BS, PT, PTT, platelets, alcohol level, toxic screen (age more than 10 years), ABGs, carbon monoxide, carboxyhemoglobin level, urinalysis
    b. Type and hold; rarely type and cross
14. Burns (second-degree, more than 30% and third-degree, more than 10%): CVP line, special lab work, cardiac monitor
15. NPO
16. Intake and output monitored
17. Analgesics (IV) preference: small dose of morphine sulfate, i.e., 5 mg q2h
18. ECG
19. O_2, 2 to 5 L/min; either mask or tongs or both
20. No steroids
21. Cover with sterile sheet
22. Consultation with inhospital staff before transferring to x-ray department and then to inpatient

on wound closure, nutritional support, and physiotherapy and occupational therapy, and, most important, when psychological support and rehabilitation activities have been initiated. Continued care starts when the acute resuscitative phase is over. This may be as soon as the patient is stabilized or when the diuresis begins. However, many elements of the acute phase may overlap aspects of continued care. For example, during diuresis, fluid management can be difficult, or the patient may require ventilatory support.

Burn wound care

In the continued care phase the prevention of invasive burn wound sepsis and the closure of the wound are emphasized, including the functional and cosmetic aspects of wound care.

The need to isolate the burn patient is always an issue: isolation can vary from sterile wound handling to complete barrier techniques.

There have been a number of studies addressing the efficacy of different types of isolator barrier systems. There are serious methodologic problems inherent in these

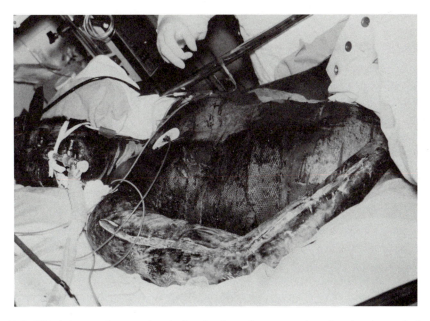

Fig. 5-4. Third-degree burns of anterior trunk and upper extremity showing subclavian venous access line and escharotomy incisions.

systems. Although the principle of preventing cross-contamination and lowering the number of bacteria in an inoculum is still valid, the primary problems are greatly depressed host resistance and infection with opportunistic organisms. These organisms are typically of such low virulence that often in the past they were considered nonpathogenic. Therefore it is not surprising that the use of isolator barrier systems has not demonstrated any superiority over standard gown, glove, and masking techniques. In addition, the difficult conditions associated with the use of an isolator barrier system add considerably to the cost and the burden of providing skilled nursing care.[9]

Fig. 5-4 demonstrates a number of issues concerning the provision of burn wound care. The patient is shown with third-degree burns of the trunk and upper extremity, with an escharotomy and placement of a subclavian venous access line penetrating through the burn wound. Although this latter access is not ideal, primarily because of the inevitable sepsis that occurs, there may be no choice because of the extent of the injured area. Similarly, some degree of cross-contamination during wound care is also inevitable in these situations. Although every effort should be made not to immerse a line site when providing wound care, there is always some contamination of the same organisms cultured from the wound. Therefore the goal should be to reduce the milieu that enhances bacterial growth by debridement of all necrotic tissue and the removal of exudate and secretions that support their growth.

In Fig. 5-4 the third-degree burn of the anterior chest wall has been grafted using a 1.5:1 Tanner-Mesh graft from the abdomen. Note that the donor sites have been left open at 24 hours following the removal of a gauze dressing impregnated with scarlet red dye in a water-soluble base, therefore allowing for open drainage and cleansing. Somewhat similarly, the grafts are also left open to provide for cleansing between the interstices of the mesh and the application of a topical antimicrobial agent.

The escharotomy on the lateral side of the upper and lower extremity, which was made shortly following admission, tends to bulge open as a result of underlying swelling. It allows for the deeper expansion of the tissues rather than compression of the circulation. The escharotomy, which should extend completely through the burn tissue to the subcutaneous tissue, but not into the fascia, results in a larger open wound which must be treated like any other open wound (i.e., cleansed and a topical antimicrobial applied).

Theoretically, although there should be no bleeding following an escharotomy through completely coagulated avascular burned skin, an occasional bleeder responds to a topical hemostatic agent such as gelfoam and, even more uncommonly, to a suture ligation. If a suture ligation is required, an absorbable suture should be used so as not to require removal or to serve as a nidus for sepsis, with a tapered needle for soft tissue and a cutting needle for hard eschar. Fairly large mattress sutures are better than simple sutures, and, unless a relatively large and isolated bleeding vessel can be identified, use of a hemostatic clamp and ligation is difficult, frustrating, and often results in rebleeding with wound care and dressing changes.

A pressure bandage is frequently of value, but proper burn care must not be neglected, particularly if the dressing is left on longer than 24 hours. Indeed, under many conditions, even for periods of time as short as 12 hours without burn wound care, the number of bacteria in the wound can increase significantly, and the occurrence of invasive burn wound sepsis can occur. Ultimately the open wound resulting from the escharotomy will require grafting like any other third-degree or full-thickness wound.

In the event the escharotomy was made in a deep second-degree but circumferential burn that compromises the circulation, the open area may epithelialize from the margins similar to any open wound. Note also that the escharotomy incision has been made along medial and lateral margins of the extremity so as not to interfere with motion by placing a restrictive scar across a flexion line.

In addition, an error in assessment may result in improper treatment, the development of burn wound sepsis and conversion to a full-thickness burn with subsequent delayed healing, increased scarring with decreased functional and cosmetic results, and, of course, increased discomfort and psychologic stress.

Care of venous access lines penetrating through burned areas can be a problem. Attending to the percutaneous site, changing at 4-day or preferably 3-day intervals, and culturing the tip of the catheter on removal will do much to prevent the

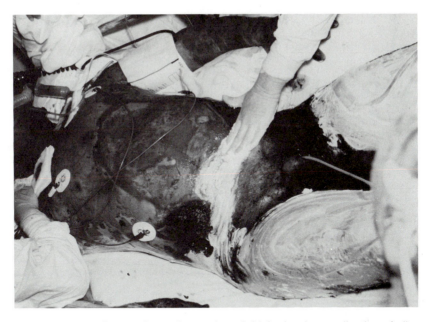

Fig. 5-5. Third-degree burns of anterior trunk and thigh showing application of silver sulfadiazine cream.

occurrence of an often confusing source of sepsis. In the event that portals of access are severely limited because of the continued need to provide for major intravenous access, the limited availability of peripheral site, or the presence of a burn wound at other usually available sites, it may be preferable to retain the present line in place.

Early grafting of hand cases, where well-defined third-degree areas or even deep second-degree areas can be identified, is highly recommended once resuscitation treatment permits safe anesthesia or even a regional nerve block. In these cases the advantages of early grafting place the hands high on the priority list for use of available skin. Although xenograft may be used if that is all that is available, it is better to use the xenograft on other less functionally critical areas of the body and use whatever autograft is available for the hands.

The application of Silvadene cream using sterile technique is shown in Fig. 5-5. The wound is first washed with an antiseptic soap and gently debrided of necrotic skin. There should be no pain or bleeding if the debridement is properly performed. *This is not the occasion for deep, full-thickness debridement.* In fact, if debridement is carried out down to and through viable tissue and if the bacterial count is high (the wound always has some level of bacteria present), an overzealous debridement may result in a shaking chill, a febrile episode, or even a major gram-negative shock syndrome.

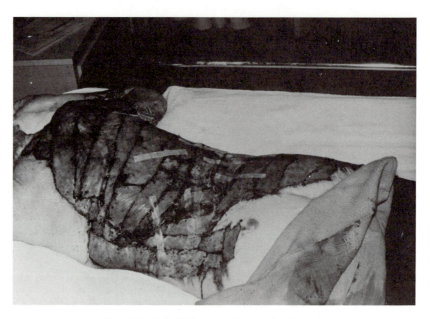

Fig. 5-6. Split-thickness skin grafts of back.

The presence or risk of a urinary tract infection with a Foley indwelling urinary catheter does not preclude the use of immersion therapy to both debride and cleanse the burn wound. If possible, however, it is preferable not to immerse any intravenous or intraarterial line. They should be protected during therapy by coverage with an antiseptic ointment at the percutaneous site, which will prevent splashed water from contaminating the wound, and by coverage with a dry sterile dressing. The dressing should be changed following the immersion, and the wound inspected.

Fig. 5-6 shows a patient with split-thickness grafts placed on a third-degree burn of the trunk. These grafts are left open, often without suturing, to facilitate daily or even twice daily debridement and cleansing. Note the exudate between even the most closely laid grafts, which can serve as bacterial media. To assist in reepithelization, it is best not to leave large spaces between the graft. Leaving large spaces makes it difficult to manage the entire wound and may accidentally destroy the grafts. If there is insufficient autograft to cover the entire wound, it is preferable to close one area completely, selecting the most critical area (e.g., over joints, tendons).

In the event of a massive burn, it is important to cover those areas in which the highest "take" is anticipated.

Another option with large open areas is the use of mesh grafts. Note the direction of grafts (see Fig. 5-6), since it can be anticipated that a scar line may very well develop along these margins and thus it is best to anticipate this event and plan the grafting in the direction of Langer's lines.

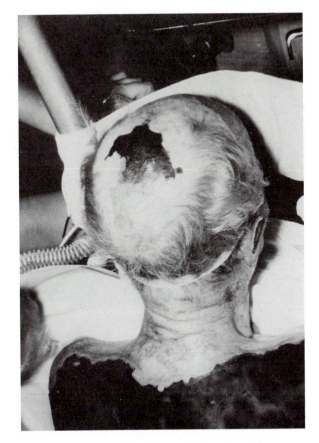

Fig. 5-7. Third-degree burn of scalp.

A patient with a third-degree burn of the scalp is shown in Fig. 5-7. This burn may have been converted by pressure from a deep second-degree burn. The patient is in the prone position with an endotracheal tube in place that is attached to a ventilator. Although this position is desirable to keep the patient from lying on the third-degree burn of the back, because of the marked decrease in thoracic compliance and resultant compromise in the ventilatory excursion it is usually not possible to place a severely burned patient in this position for very long. Similarly, the use of rotating frames is usually not possible because of the same ventilatory constraint.

Whether to debride bullae is often a question. Although early removal prevents the collection of an exudate rich in bacterial nutrients, retention is more comfortable and may prevent the wound from drying out with subsequent discomfort and may prevent injury to any remaining viable epithelial cells. Bullae also provide a temporary barrier to invasive bacteria. The recommended treatment, therefore, is careful cleansing of the wound followed by application of a topical antimicrobial agent and

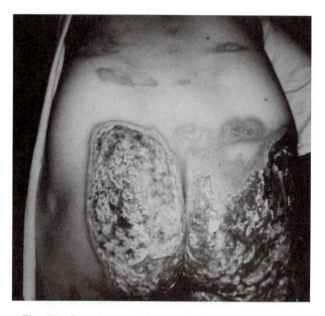

Fig. 5-8. Deep second-degree flame burn of buttocks.

preservation of the intact bullae. If the bullae have been ruptured, but are otherwise intact, then it is recommended that they be retained in place at least for the first several days, taking care to cleanse them carefully and to debride earlier than otherwise indicated.

In any case, the wound must be inspected at least daily, and at the earliest sign of any cloudy collection or erythema, the bullae should be completely debrided, the wound and the fluid cultured, and the newly exposed wound treated promptly with an antibacterial agent. If the wound can be kept free from bacterial invasion, the bullae usually break during the cleansing process or accidentally with pressure about the fifth to seventh day postburn and thereafter expose a second-degree wound with thin but pink healing epithelium.

Where the skin is very thick, such as on the dorsum of the hand or sole of the foot, the bullae may need to be incised and debrided at this time.

Fig. 5-8 shows a deep second-degree burn of the buttocks that was treated in 1964 just following the introduction of sulfamylon, the first effective method to control burn wound sepsis. Before this time, treatment would have consisted of a diverting colostomy and the inevitable occurrence of burn wound sepsis, resulting in a conversion to a third-degree burn. In these instances the surgeon would have been unaware that the wound was only deep second in the beginning. One of the reasons for this lack of awareness is that the epithelium in deep hair follicles can reepithelize a wound if these fragile cells are not destroyed by infection, pressure, or the application of toxic agents such as tannic or picric acid.

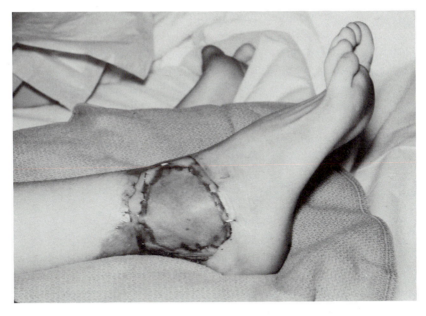

Fig. 5-9. Split-thickness graft 5 days after applications.

A patient with a third-degree burn of the ankle with split-thickness skin graft clipped in place is shown in Fig. 5-9. The graft overlaps the wound margin. This type of complete closure, i.e., without "pie crusting" or drainage incisions, can only be applied on a healthy granulating base with a low bacterial count. The wound must be inspected daily so that an unsuspected area of undebrided necrosis or septic nidus can be drained or debrided before it spreads underneath and causes the entire graft to slough. Early removal of alternating clips also helps to facilitate "milking" of underlying serum or exudate, the continued presence of which serves as a focus for infection.

Pulmonary support

Although active ventilatory support may extend into the continued care phase, the main objective of pulmonary support in the continued care phase is the treatment or the prevention of sepsis. Opportunistic organisms of low virulence frequently inhabit the respiratory tract, requiring intensive and continued attention to pulmonary toilet, regular sputum cultures, and the use of sterile technique to reduce the size of the inevitable inoculum that occurs with repeated suctioning.

In the event that a tracheostomy was necessary, even more meticulous attention to the details of sterile technique is required. Three main problems exist in reducing the possibility of sepsis:

1. The enhancement of the normal host defense mechanisms, such as with optimal nutritional support, and the decreased use of those drugs that depress host resistance
2. The reduction in the material within the bronchial tree that provides the nutritional media for bacterial growth
3. The reduction in both type and amount of the constant inoculum associated with bronchial cleaning regimens, and the frequent removal of bronchial exudate from bacterial growth and presence of white cells followed by identification of specific treatment when indicated

The constant use of broad-spectrum antibiotics on a prophylactic basis has little value except in crisis situations wherein the patient is doing poorly, there is every indication which antibiotic is required, and time does not permit specific identification and sensitivity testing.

The antibiotics usually indicated for these low-virulence, opportunistic organism situations are often those of high toxicity and rapid sensitization. Guidelines require balancing the clinical situation with renal function and serum levels. These assessments are mandatory, either by measuring the levels of the specific agent or, if not possible, measuring those indications of toxicity such as BUN, creatinine, and liver function. Daily monitoring of the bacterial flora is also required.

The current problem is not only treating for long periods of time (i.e., over 10 days) but changing prescriptions too soon; an antibiotic, once indicated, should not be changed under 5 days unless toxicity ensues or some specific new data become available.

Fever in burn patients is not unusual despite long-term antibiotic usage. If a clinical appraisal does not indicate the source of a low-grade fever, the antibiotics should be stopped, and the situation reappraised.

The temperature of the patient with major burn injury may be 1° or 2° F ($-16°$ or $-17°$ C) above normal temperature as a result of hypermetabolism, or more insidious, subnormal (97° or 98° F; 36° to 37° C), with severe sepsis caused by insensible water loss with its obligatory energy requirement, the presence of a gram-negative infection, or the use of antipyretics.

The question of how long an endotracheal tube can be left in place without the development of pressure necrosis of the larynx brings into consideration the pros and cons of the alternate, usually tracheostomy vs. extubation. A comparison of the advantages and disadvantages of tracheostomy, nasotracheal airway, and oropharyngeal airway are listed in Table 5-2.

Nutritional support

Three developments in the past 30 years have resulted in as much as an 80% reduction in mortality of the patients with a major burn injury: improvement in hemodynamic and ventilatory management, control of burn wound sepsis, and improved nutritional support.[3,27,32,43]

Table 5-2. Tracheostomy vs. nasopharyngeal/oropharyngeal airway*

	Tracheostomy	Nasopharyngeal	Oropharyngeal
Ease of insertion	+	+ +	+ + +
Pulmonary sepsis	100%†	+	+
Pulmonary toilet	+ +	+	+
Patient comfort	+ +	+ +	+
Ventilation efficiency	+ + +	+ + +	+ + +
Laryngeal scarring	+	+ +	+ +
Duration acceptable	N/A‡	2 weeks	3 weeks

*+, ++, +++ indicate increasing subjective or objective, though immeasurable, probability.
†All burn patients with a tracheostomy acquire pulmonary sepsis, the greater majority to a severe degree, as opposed to those treated with either a nasopharyngeal or an oropharyngeal tracheal tube in whom pulmonary sepsis is frequently, but not uniformly, a major complication.
‡The duration that endotracheal tubes can be used without the need for sedation and without the laryngeal scarring or severe sepsis has gradually increased with better tubes and better management. At present, endotracheal tubes can be used even up to 6 weeks. The nasopharyngeal/oropharyngeal tube can be used even longer and usually is preferable to the complications of an early tracheostomy.

Success with the resuscitation or shock phase led to patients dying later of burn wound sepsis. Improvement in the control of burn wound sepsis resulted in patients still dying of sepsis, but of pulmonary rather than wound sepsis and of sepsis caused by less virulent organisms. The implementation of nutritional programs has resulted in the preservation and/or restoration of the body's host defense mechanisms, therefore greatly reducing the chance of dying from a low-virulent, opportunistic organism. This has been clearly shown both clinically and in laboratory animals. Refinements continue in the entire field of nutritional support, but of particular interest are those aspects that have application to patients with thermal injury.

Indications. Several basic principles must be considered in deciding who should receive nutritional support, when, in what form, and to what degree.

All burn patients admitted should be evaluated for the possibility of nutritional support. These include the critically burned patient (i.e., an adult who has a second- or third-degree burn greater than 20% total BSA, a child who has a second- or third-degree burn of 10% total BSA), as well as those with minor injuries. Evidence increasingly indicates the need to support patients with smaller burns. Perhaps this approach reflects the increasing awareness that large segments of the population, especially among those in the injury-prone group, have marginal nutritional status.

It is essential to start these nutritional programs before there is any noticeable depletion such as weight loss. To play catch-up is exceedingly difficult and fraught with failure.

Because of hemodynamic complications, it is difficult to institute a program during the resuscitative phase before 5 days postburn. At this point diuresis has usually started, and, although it will take several days to get the nutritional support up to full amount, this slight delay is not significant. There may also be a delay in attaining the full support during this period, either parenterally because of complications such as hyperglycemia or enterally because of ileus or diarrhea. What is important is the inclusion of the nutritional support team in the early planning stage.

Metabolic response. It was recognized in the early 1960s that a hypermetabolism as much as two times normal in patients with a major thermal injury results in a protein loss that can cause muscle wasting, immunosuppression, impaired wound healing, and increased bacterial susceptibility and death within a few weeks.[19,40] The patients actually starve to death.

Wilmore[46] showed that this postburn elevation of the metabolic rate is in proportion to the size of the thermal injury and reaches a maximum in patients with a burn wound of 50% to 60% total BSA. He also demonstrated that these rates do not return to normal until the wound is completely closed.

Although there has been considerable research regarding relationship of insensible water loss and the obligatory energy loss with evaporation, it is now accepted that this loss is not the primary reason for the hypermetabolic state. The hypermetabolic rate is temperature sensitive, however, but not temperature dependent. Thus the application of external heat or the prevention of insensible water loss through the skin will not eliminate the hypermetabolic state. Nevertheless, the neglect of these aspects will aggravate the situation.

With respect to the hypermetabolic response in burn patients, the following aspects should be considered in providing nutritional support:

1. Oxygen consumption will be near normal during the emergent resuscitative phase but will be followed by rises and peaks in the presence of infection or stressful operations.
2. There is an increase in water loss as a result of increased hormonal release.
3. Catecholamines—the evidence suggests that increased catecholamines and adrenergic activity are the major cholinergic mediators responsible for the hypermetabolic response following injury.[12]
4. Glucose—glucose kinetics are also altered following injury, and the glucose tolerance and insulin responses are dampened. This must be addressed on an individual basis.[45]
5. Nitrogen—a marked loss of nitrogen results from increased use of protein for calories. Amino acids, particularly alanine, are released and converted to glucose, providing readily available fuel for glucose-dependent tissues.

Requirements

Calories. In 1974, Curreri and associates[11] proposed a formula to estimate caloric requirements according to body weight and burn size. A problem with its application, like that of its predecessor, the Harris-Benedict equation, is that it does not account for rapid fluctuations and leads to weight gain. It is widely used and is more practical clinically than the measurements of metabolic rates, although bedside indirect calorimetry is now feasible and worthwhile in difficult cases or as an occasional check on the adequacy of nutritional replacement.[4]

Indirect calorimetry is based on the fact that all metabolic processes are oxidative processes.[11,36]

Using these methods, the respiratory quotient (RQ) can be evaluated clinically. Therefore an RQ of 0.85 is indicative of "mixed substrate oxidation" and is seen in patients who are well-nourished, whereas clinically an RQ over 1 suggests fat synthesis and overfeeding, and conversely an RQ of 0.7 or below is found in patients at starvation level.

Daily caloric requirements for adults and children calculated according to Curreri in 1974 (and verified in 1985) are as follows[11,16]:

$$\text{Curreri: Adults: } (25 \times \text{wt[kg]}) + (40 \times \text{total BSA})$$
$$\text{Children: } (60 \times \text{wt[kg]}) + (35 \times \text{total BSA})$$

A number of studies have shown that, when patient caloric requirements are met, the optimum protein sparing effect occurs if 15% to 25% are administered as protein rather than glucose or lipid.

Protein. In addition to the usual essential amino acids, the nutritional support should be augmented by cysteine, arginine, and histidine. In this regard, Alexander and associates[1] have reported that whey products provide cysteine, since hypocysteinemia occurs frequently in burned children. Similar to cysteine, arginine in burn patients is not synthesized in adequate amounts from the normal urea cycle and should be added. It has been difficult to prove clinically, but a 2% arginine supplementation has been shown to be beneficial in guinea pigs. The need for additional histidine is not as clear as that for cysteine and arginine, but it appears that additional amounts are beneficial.

Lipids. Lipids are required because of the need for wound healing, cellular integrity, and absorption of fat-soluble vitamins, but extra fat results in complications such as cholestasis, hepatomegaly, impaired clotting, and decreased resistance to infection.

It has been demonstrated that fat infusion resulted in no protein sparing effect in burn patients. Glucose in burn patients is a more efficient energy source than fat. It is recommended, however, that 20% to 25% of the caloric requirement can be supplied by lipid infusion.

Micronutrients. The recommended dietary allowances should be given rather than an overall increased requirement for all of these substances; there is no indication that megadoses are of value.

Water. Sufficient water should be given to replace insensible loss. This is discussed in detail in Chapter 6 under problems such as hypernatremia.

Insulin. Following a burn injury, patients are often hyperglycemic and demonstrate glucose intolerance—an exaggerated insulin response may also occur and further confound management.[6]

Energy support. In summary, there are a number of adages that can be applied to ensure that the burn victim receives maximum energy or nutritional support. Among these is the need to reduce metabolic stress through reduction of insensible water loss and to maintain optimum environmental temperature; the need to start support early before deterioration occurs to carefully assess the requirement; the awareness that overfeeding is not beneficial and that hyperalimentation produces an often difficult to manage hyperglycemia; the recognition that the safest route is enteral, using either oral or tube feeding with constant infusion; finally, the recognition that complications such as diarrhea, fever, and retention of tubes and lines require innovative and persistent attention to succeed.

Nursing services

The nurse is particularly concerned with coordination and supervision of the overall management of the total care of the burn patient. Although nurses' first priorities are often subsumed by disciplines such as respiratory therapy, nutritional support teams, and physiotherapy or occupational therapy, the daily care of the burn wound, nutritional support, pain control, and the psychosocial adjustment, including family relationships, are in the nurse's domain.

Pain control. Pain control is often a problem.[24,42] There is frequently a fear of oversedation and/or developing addiction, despite data to the contrary. In a study reported by Porter and Jack[34] in 1980, of 11,882 patients receiving narcotics for pain control, primarily for maintaining patient comfort and to ensure treatment cooperation, the addiction rate was only 0.1%. It has also been reported that once the wound is closed, there is a dramatic reduction in the need for analgesics. In order to provide the most comfort, it is essential that a protocol for administering pain medication be established, with the nurse being identified as the coordinator.

Generally, smaller and more frequent doses are preferable, with morphine being the most common, followed by meperidine and codeine. The judicious use of small doses of psychotropics can also be of benefit. It is critical to design a program whereby pain medication is administered to allow the patient to perform such activities of daily living as resting, bathing, and ambulating.

The assessment of pain can be difficult; in most treatment settings the nurse is in the best position to assess pain. There are, however, some objective guidelines that can be used to evaluate pain such as location and degree of the burn; alterations in physiologic or behavioral parameters, particularly in response to medication; and the patient's description and response to activities such as ambulation, bathing, debridement, and dressing change.

There are a number of rating measures for evaluating pain, including the often used method of having the patient rate pain intensity on a numeric scale (e.g., 1 to 10). Together with the nurse assessments, these can be helpful in developing a strategy for treating the patient and, very often, the patient's family.

The route of the administration of the analgesic can be a problem in a severely burned patient. If an IV is already in place, a pain-free injection route with a rapid response time is thus available, which is of value not only in quickly reducing the pain, but in assessing the pain management. The intramuscular (IM) or subcutaneous (SC) route can be a problem because of lack of suitable sites, and it is often because of this that the oral route, the most desirable in long-term care, is used without a transition from IV through IM to p.o. With p.o. medication, a different dose equivalency, timing, and absorption rate must be considered. The use of suppositories in situations with limited IV access and absorption or cooperation problems can be invaluable even for morphine, but the absorption amount and rate may vary considerably.

Education and training. It is essential that the burn nurse play a role in the education and training of nursing personnel; physiotherapists and respiratory and occupational therapists; dieticians; and social workers, who may have had little or no contact with the care of patients with a thermal injury. This training extends to medical students and residents; nursing students; and the patients and their families, to augment hospital care such as in the areas of physiotherapy and nutritional support and, most important, on the psychosocial level. The patient and family must come to a point at which they have acquired the skills to continue the treatment on an outpatient basis.[5]

Physiotherapy and occupational therapy

Considerable overlap exists between the functions of the physiotherapist and occupational therapist in the treatment of burn patients, which will vary between institutions and interests.[21-23,33]

The involvement of these disciplines in the development of a comprehensive program of positioning, splinting, exercise, ambulation, and the activities of daily living should be accomplished within 24 hours following burn injury.

The physiotherapy and occupational therapy appraisal has as its goal a plan to attain the maximum restoration of optimal level of function at the earliest possible time. To achieve this goal, there must be close communication and cooperation between all the professionals involved through conferences and agreement concerning evaluations and goals.

The early involvement of physiotherapy and the frequent use of both active and passive motion is a rehabilitation imperative. Actual physiotherapy should start as soon as the patient is able to start active motion or at least passive motion and the use of splints to reduce the possibility of contractures. In practice, both active and passive motion are difficult during the acute edema phase, but, if instituted during these days, they do start the patient on a rehabilitation "fast track," particularly from a psychologic perspective.

One critical constraining factor in these rehabilitation efforts is the need to prevent a burn wound sepsis that invades or inflames the tendon sheaths, the ligaments, and the joints and joint capsules, resulting in scarring and adhesions that severely restrict motion. Thus use of a splint that acts as an occlusive dressing that may enhance bacterial growth or pressure necrosis may hamper efforts to pay attention to meticulous wound care. This concern can be best overcome by (1) providing a smooth, well-fitting splint without rough spots, well padded with absorbable dressing, between any nonabsorbable surface such as the splint itself or (2) the use of a foam padding; frequent, even twice daily removal and dressing or padding changes; and the early use of cleansing and debriding hydrotherapy.

Pain is often a severe deterrent to the inexperienced therapist; careful coordination of the patient's pain medication with other activities and with hydrotherapy for cleansing and debridement is required. Often the family can least understand causing the patient more pain; therefore it is critical to gain their support and help them understand the necessity for early physiotherapy. Including the family in decisions also helps them to adjust to the patient's condition and prepares them for actually providing the continued care within the hospital and thereafter on an outpatient basis following hospitalization.

The use of innovative splints and prosthetic devices on the basis of sound principles of wound care are important challenges (i.e., arm hammocks for elevation of the thermally injured upper extremity, netting leg supports for circumferential burns that allow for drying and drainage, adaptations of thermoplastic and foam devices that evenly distribute skin pressure, and the use of dynamic splints that enhance motion).

Planning for continued care

Planning for continued care, both within the hospital and in the home setting, begins the day of admission, including coordination and scheduling of hospital services such as the aforementioned physiotherapy and occupational therapy, surgical debridement, wound closure, and reconstruction schedules.

The factors to be considered in planning surgical procedures on patients with a major thermal injury are as follows:

1. Overall prognosis and goals
2. Patient condition
   a. Hemodynamic and respiratory status
   b. Hepatic and renal function
   c. Nutritional status
3. Wound status
   a. Amount of debridement required
   b. Number and type of bacterial growth
   c. Amount of autograft or other wound coverage

4. Operating and recovery room
   a. Type and duration of anesthesia
   b. Skill and number of personnel
   c. Equipment and temperature
5. Availability of blood transfusions

Each item has been discussed elsewhere, but during the periodic planning meetings these factors are reviewed in detail.

Discharge planning includes locating the patient's residence, providing professional supervision and treatment, revising the home for support of the disabled patient (i.e., safety rails, hospital beds, wheelchairs, and ramps), and making arrangements necessary for financial coverage. Very often, nothing is more beneficial to the patient's morale than the knowledge that sufficient funds are available to provide for both patient and family care.

The establishment of a schedule for each patient showing the location and the event (e.g., laboratory tests, physiotherapy, debridement, or discharge) will do much to coordinate the team activities, as well as give the patient actual goals upon which he may establish beneficial patterns.

Medical records and diagnosis related groups

Complete medical records have long been recognized as essential to providing and continuing care and reviewing and appraising the patient's progress. It is becoming increasingly important to keep medical records, including diagnosis and procedures that facilitate third-party reviews and compensation. From a practical and ethical viewpoint, the care of the patient with thermal injuries is often associated with legal liability, either civil or criminal, compensation, and high costs. Therefore, in the best interest of the patients, the health care facilities and providers, and those involved in research, teaching, and prevention, these records should be complete.

Diagnosis Related Groups (DRGs) are the basis of Medicare's hospital reimbursement program, which provides a means of relating the type of patients that a hospital treats (i.e., case mix) to the costs incurred by the hospital.[10,30,39]

Using this system, a patient is assigned a DRG based on clinical information from the patient's medical record, primarily the discharge summary and the face sheet, rather than the progress notes. Medical record personnel examine the medical record, assigning diagnosis codes and extracting data elements that are the basis for determining the DRG. A computer program called "GROUPER" applies a decision tree to the extracted clinical information in order to assign the DRG.

The physician's role is to be precise and detailed in listing the clinical information. The types of information used to calculate the DRG are:
1. The principal diagnosis, which is established after evaluation, rather than the admitting diagnosis

2. The secondary diagnosis, which is the condition existing at the time of admission or as a result of subsequent developments or complications that affect treatment received and/or length of stay (This information is critical to justify situations in which the patient's stay is longer and/or more costly to the hospital than the norm.)

3. The principal procedure performed for definitive treatment rather than for diagnostic or exploratory purposes or that was necessary to take care of a complication during the hospitalization

4. Age of the patient expressed in years

5. Sex of the patient

6. Discharge status, the circumstances under which the patient left the hospital
   a. Routine discharge to home
   b. Discharge against medical advice
   c. Transferred
   d. Expired

When considering the format for detailing the diagnosis, the physician should proceed as follows:

1. List the principal diagnosis first. The order of any multiple secondary diagnoses is not critical because the GROUPER software will rank them. However, the physician must identify the principal diagnosis.

2. Describe the diagnosis using the nomenclature of the International Classification of Diseases, revision 9, Clinical Modifications (ICD-9-CM), because this is the coding system used by medical record personnel.

3. Be familiar with the structure of ICD-9-CM codes for burns. Burns are coded within the range of 940 to 948. They are classified according to site (multiple is its own code), extent of burn (BSA), and depth of burn (first-, second-, or third-degree). The coding structure allows for specificity concerning total BSA and the percentage of BSA involving a third-degree burn, if any.

The following are guidelines to use in writing face sheets and discharge summaries:

1. List the highest degree burn first. When there are different degrees of burns in the same site, identify the highest degree as the principal diagnosis.

2. Indicate the existence of any infection in the burn site or any other complications as a secondary diagnosis. In particular, clearly identify any infected wound sites.

3. List all procedures such as debridements, grafting, intubations, or long-line insertions occurring during the hospital stay.

4. Identify the percentage of total BSA burned and associate it with the depth of burn. In third-degree burns, if no body surface area was involved, it should also be noted.

5. List the cause of burn ("E" codes).

6. Avoid writing, "Burn, unspecified" or any vague or incomplete description that would prevent a coder from entering the most specific data possible.

7. Be prepared to provide a comprehensive discharge summary and copies of operative procedures or any documentation, including photographs or burn charts, that may be requested.
8. Since DRG payments are based on the average costs, complete medical documentation is the best basis for appeals.

OUTPATIENT CARE

Outpatient care includes all care the patient receives once he or she leaves the hospital. In the past only patients with the most minor burn or the major burn patients in whom all wounds were closed and whose only reason for return to the acute level facility was for reconstruction or cosmetic surgery received outpatient care.

With the emergence of extensive home care support resources, rehabilitation hospitalization, and increased financial costs, and, most of all, with the recognition that patients generally do better psychologically, and even physiologically, in their home environment, patients are now being discharged with open wounds awaiting further debridement and grafting.

Therefore home care now includes many facets heretofore limited to the hospital and critical to the success of the rehabilitation. Planning must include hospital personnel, the family, upon whom much of the care will fall, and the members of the home health agency who very likely are unfamiliar with many aspects of burn care. These concerns largely fall into the following areas: burn wound care, physiotherapy, nutritional support, psychologic and social adjustment, and financial management.

Thus many aspects discussed under the continued care section also apply to outpatient care. However, it is critical to address the need for reassurance to the patient, family, and most especially the various health providers. Since it is evident that a viable home care program is not achieved by good intentions per se, active education and training sessions are a prerequisite. There is a need to recognize the effect of stress on the family members, both within the hospital setting and at home.

Although it has been shown that 85% of patients with major burns (i.e., over 30% total BSA) attained a full restoration of social adjustment, it should be emphasized to the family and the patient that this restoration of social function takes at least 1 year following the injury to even fully assess.

Burn wound care

Home treatment of the patient with an open wound should be similar to that received in the hospital. However, there are several differences: at home, sterile procedures are difficult. Emphasis should be on such factors as clean technique, frequent hand-washing by all personnel, use of clean linen, and towels. Laundering with detergent and a hot water wash or rinse, in a washing machine, or washing dishes in a dishwasher or a 180° F (82.2° C) hot water rinse will normally create sterile conditions. The patient must be protected from infected visitors, i.e., from those with upper respiratory infections or other systemic or skin conditions, to protect not only the wound but also the patient whose resistance may be compromised by the burn injury.

Cleansing. Use of an ordinary shower or bathtub is acceptable, providing the tub is washed in normal fashion and the room is kept warm and free from drafts that may chill the patient. Detergent soaps are also of benefit in removing exudate and reducing the bacterial count, but actually any soap will function in this capacity, and it is desirable to select one that is acceptable to the patient. Antiseptic washes such as betadine soap are generally not aesthetically desirable or necessary unless specifically indicated. Family members may need to be reminded that the burn patient with an open wound harbors no exotic germs but only those of very low virulence, which are usually only pathogenic in a patient with a severely depressed host defense mechanism and certainly are no threat to the family.

Similarly, perfumed soaps and hair shampoos will not harm the wound and are often psychologically of great benefit to the patient. But if there is a stinging sensation with the use of any of these products, an extra effort should be made to thoroughly rinse the wounds. Burned patients are often hypersensitive to either hot or cold water, and, although warmer water may provide more thorough cleansing, the actual temperature is irrelevant compared to patient comfort.

Open wounds. Open wounds are frequently treated with topical antimicrobial agents at home. In the interest of providing the "best care," they are often applied too frequently, and an intense effort is made to keep some of the agent on the wound at all times. Family and patients need to be instructed as to the proper frequency and dosage (i.e., applications three to four times per day are usually sufficient).

They should also be reassured that all linen and clothing that has contact with these agents can be cleansed in an ordinary washing machine. Simple, inexpensive cotton underwear, shirts, pants, and socks should be purchased. Moreover, loose-fitting clothing is more comfortable; for example, suspenders can be preferable to a belt. Patients usually feel better if they are well-groomed and dressed each day.

Grooming should include haircuts, shaves, and the use of cosmetics, together with professional hairdressing and all the other adjuvants that enhance the patient's feeling of well-being.

There is often a fear of an open wound, particularly if occasional spotting or bleeding occurs, and a tendency to cover all wounds or to place numerous ointments or creams on the wound, often of the home remedy type. Constant reassurance in these circumstances is necessary to ensure compliance with the prescribed treatment modality. The use of nonadherent dressings that do not allow for the absorption of exudate is also to be condemned.

The presence of an eschar is somewhat more comfortable, but the patient and the family need to be instructed on its gradual sloughing or debridement. The more

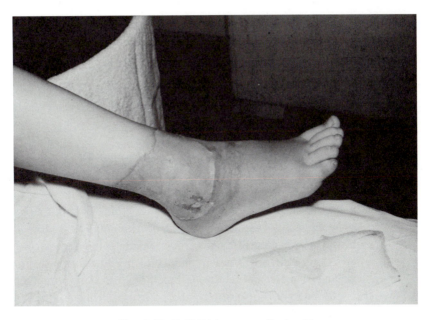

Fig. 5-10. Split-thickness graft of ankle.

instruction the family receives, the better the care of the patient will be. Above all, nothing replaces a home visit by a knowledgeable professional to allay fear and to ensure compliance.

Temperature in the house is often a concern because of the fear of catching cold. Patients require and are most comfortable in temperatures in which they do not shiver, since shivering requires the use of more energy. Often a humidifier is of benefit, particularly if there has been an inhalation injury.

Closed wounds. Reepithelized or grafted skin areas are less sensitive, thin, and easily subjected to trauma. These areas must be protected from chaffing by clothing or injury. An example of a problem area is shown in Fig. 5-10, which shows a split-thickness graft of the anterior ankle, for which a soft dressing and soft slippers are desirable. Elastic stockings or bandages are beneficial when swelling occurs, but extraordinary care should be taken with their use to prevent pressure ulceration. A good, smooth fit, sometimes over a cotton absorbent stocking, and daily inspections and cleaning are mandatory.

Itching, a tight or restrictive feeling, and dryness are frequent problems that can be managed by using a nongreasy water-soluble base lotion or cream such as lanolin. In actual practice a number of commercially available skin lotions and hand creams are usually more acceptable to the patient than plain lanolin. For severe urticaria, a steroid-containing cream may be of benefit. Hormones or vitamin additives are costly and have not been shown to have any benefit.

Elastic garments, usually specifically fitted, have been shown to be helpful in reducing scar formation and are recommended, again taking care that the easily damaged, underlying thin skin not be abraded.

Clothing selected to cover disfigured areas may help the patient adjust better. The importance of body image cannot be overstressed, although it has been shown that many other aspects of the spousal relationship are more critical to acceptance and support.

Physiotherapy

Physiotherapy and occupational therapy start in the resuscitative phase, extend through the hospitalization period, and continue into outpatient care. During this time the intensity of the activity will vary, depending on continued assessment. A full appraisal is indicated just before and shortly following discharge. This should include careful functional measurements in coordination with the treating physician, the setting of goals, and selection of methods and initiation of a program of supervision and support. Education of the patient and his support network or family is essential to success. Discussion of the facilities at home, especially if augmented by a home visit, will do much to ensure success. Finally, cooperation with a work or educational program to enable completion of school programs or the acquisition of new skills that permit the patient to reenter the work force will do much to rehabilitate the patient.

Most people with major burns are admitted to hospitals and therefore more easily enter the health system and have the opportunity to receive physiotherapy or occupational therapy; the patient with the minor burn often does not receive this therapy. Functional loss and delay in returning to full productivity are difficult to determine, but it is clear that all patients with even minor involvement with critical functional areas such as hands should be evaluated for possible therapy.

Nutritional support

All patients hospitalized with major thermal injury require some level of nutritional support following discharge. To be effective, the program must be discussed in conference with the dietician, the patient, and, most important, the family members who shop and prepare the food. In this regard, there are several specific areas that must be addressed. A follow-up conference is beneficial if the support is to be optimum.[29]

1. Patients are being discharged early and at a stage that may still require intensive nutritional support.
2. Preburn nutrition status and habits may have been marginal because of lack of knowledge or motivation, cultural or financial.
3. A postburn home nutrition program must take into account all of the preburn factors in addition to cultural and preburn dietary habits.

4. Numerous questions should be anticipated regarding the benefits of special diets, additives, and vitamins.

Psychologic and social adjustment

The ultimate goal of all burn care is not only patient survival but a successful continuation of life. Several maxims impact on the probability of success: patients with adjustment problems before burn injury will still have problems (e.g., school adjustment, behavioral problems such as alcohol or other substance abuse, poor work history, elderly with minimal social support that affects the elderly, physical or mental deficits, or adverse financial status affecting all groups). These prior conditions are added to those incurred by the thermal injury; all patients with a major burn require evaluation and some level of support. Many of those with minor burns also require an appraisal and often some level of support either because of physical, cosmetic, or social issues associated with the injury or because the injury has presented an opportunity to identify other issues that need to be addressed such as child abuse.[8,28]

There are a number of support groups that have been formed throughout the country aimed toward the patient or his family. Although access is most readily secured through admission to a burn center, they are also available to patients treated at other facilities.

The contact should be made early, either through a social service department or by calling a burn center. These support groups have usually been started by former burn injury patients or their families and work closely with professional burn care providers.[7,31,35,38]

REFERENCES

1. Alexander, JW, et al: Beneficial effects of aggressive protein feeding in severely burned children, Ann Surg 192:505, 1980.
2. Allyn, P, and Bartlett, R: Management of the burn patient. In Zschoche, DA, editor: Comprehensive review of critical care, St. Louis, 1981, The CV Mosby Co.
3. Aulich, LH, et al: The relative significance of thermal and metabolic demands on burn hypermetabolism, J Trauma 19:559, 1979.
4. Bartlett, RH, et al: Nutritional therapy based on positive caloric balance in burned patients, Arch Surg 112:974, 1972.
5. Bayley, EW: Nursing education in a burn unit, Crit Care Quart 7:63, 1984.
6. Black, PR, et al: Mechanisms of insulin resistance following injury, Ann Surg 196:420, 1983.
7. Blades, BC, Jones, C, and Munster, AM: Quality of life after burn injuries, J Trauma 19:557, 1979.
8. Bryne, C, et al: The social competence of children following burn injury: A study of resilience, J Burn Care Rehabil 7:247, 1986.
9. Choctaw, WT: Is there a need for barrier isolators with laminar air flow in managing adult patients with major burns, J Burn Care Rehabil 5:331, 1984.
10. Converse, M, editor: Coding clinic for ICD-9-CM, Chicago, 1984-1986, AMA Div of Quality Management.
11. Curreri, PW, et al: Dietary requirements of patients with major burns, J Am Diet Assn 65:415, 1974.
12. Davies, CL, et al: The relationship of increased oxygen consumption to catecholamine excretion in thermal burns, Ann Surg 165:169, 1967.

13. Diller, KR, Hayes, LJ, and Baxter, CR: A mathematical model for the thermal efficacy of cooling therapy for burns, J Burn Care 4:81, 1983.
14. Dunham, CM, and Lamonica, C: Prolonged tracheal intubation in the trauma patient, J Trauma 24:120, 1984.
15. Durtschi, MB, et al: A prospective study of prophylactic penicillin in acutely burned hospitalized patients, J Trauma 22:11, 1982.
16. Dyess, DL, et al: The Curreri formula revisited, Proc Am Burn Assn (abstr 31) 17:31, 1985.
17. Frank, HA, and Wachtel, TL: Life and death in a burn center, J Burn Care 5:339, 1984.
18. Gordon, M, editor: Burn care protocols for nutritional support, J Burn Care Rehabil 7: 351, 1986.
19. Gump, FE, and Kinney, JM: Energy balance and weight loss in burned patients, Arch Surg 103:442, 1972.
20. Hill, MB, Achauer, BM, and Martinez, S: Tar and asphalt burns, J Burn Care 5:271, 1984.
21. Johnson, C: PT/OT forum, J Burn Care Rehabil 7:148, 1986.
22. Johnson, C: PT/OT forum, J Burn Care Rehabil 7:266, 1986.
23. Johnson, C: PT/OT forum, J Burn Care Rehabil 8:56, 1987.
24. Kibbee, E: Burn pain management, Crit Care Quart 7:54, 1984.
25. Knudson-Cooper, M: What are the research priorities in the behavioral areas for burn patients? J Trauma 24:S197, 1984.
26. Leonard, LG, Scheulen, JJ, and Munster, AM: Chemical burns: effect of prompt first aid, J Trauma 22:420, 1982.
27. Lescher, TJ, Sirinek, KR, and Pruitt, BA, Jr: Superior mesenteric artery syndrome in thermally injured patients, J Trauma 19:567, 1979.
28. Manger, G, and Speed, E: A coordinated approach to discharge of burned children, J Burn Care Rehabil 7:127, 1986.
29. Manning, SE, Hedberg, AM, and Beesinger, DE: A nutritional audit: process and product, J Burn Care 3:371, 1982.
30. Marvin, J: Burn care update: burn nursing and DRG reimbursement, J Burn Care Rehabil 5:319, 1984.
31. Mitchell, JT, and Resnik, HLP: Emergency response to crisis, Bowie, Md, 1981, Robert J. Brady Co.
32. Moratz, MA, et al: Clinical values of the prognostic nutritional index in burn patients, J Burn Care 5:294, 1984.
33. Nadel, E, and Kozerefski, PM: Rehabilitation of the critically ill burn patient, Crit Care Quart 7:19, 1984.
34. Porter, I, and Jack, H: Addiction rate in patients treated with narcotics, N Engl J Med 302:123, 1980.
35. Reddish, A, and Blumenfield, M: Psychological reactions in wives of patients with severe burns, J Burn Care 5:388, 1984.
36. Saffle, JR, et al: Use of indirect calorimetry in the nutritional management of burned patients, J Trauma 25:32, 1985.
37. Saydari, R, et al: Chemical burns, J Burn Care Rehabil 7:404, 1986.
38. Schiller, WR: Tar burns in the southwest, Surg Gynecol Obstet 157:38, 1983.
39. Silverstein, P, et al: Round table discussion— The advent of prospective payment: how DRG's could affect burn centers, J Burn Care 5:301, 1984.
40. Soroff, HS, Pearson, E, and Artz, CP: An evaluation of nitrogen requirements for equilibrium in burn patients, Surg Gynecol Obstet 112:159, 1961.
41. Stinnett, JD, et al: Plasma and skeletal muscle amino acids following severe burn injury in patients and experimental animals, Ann Surg 195:75, 1985.
42. Torgerson, WS: What objective measures are there for evaluating pain? J Trauma 24:S187, 1984.
43. Vaughan, GM, et al: Cortisol and corticotropin in burned patients, J Trauma 22:263, 1982.
44. Wachtel, TL, Parks, SN, and Dimick, AR: Early enzymatic debridement and grafting of burned hands: evaluating the travase fast-graft method in deep dermal burns, J Burn Care 5:325, 1983.
45. Wilmore, DW, Mason, AD, Jr, and Pruitt, BA, Jr: Impaired glucose flow in burned patients with gram-negative sepsis, Surg Gynecol Obstet 183:314, 1976.
46. Wilmore, DW, et al: Catecholamines: mediators of the hypermetabolic response to thermal injury, Ann Surg 180:653, 1974.
47. Young, VR, Motil, KJ, and Burke, JF: Energy and protein metabolism in relation to requirements of burned pediatric patients. In Suskind, RM, editor: Textbook of pediatric nutrition, New York, 1981, Raven Press.

6 Fluid Therapy

PRINCIPLES OF FLUID THERAPY
Overview

Recognition of the huge fluid losses and the need for adequate replacement following a major thermal injury has contributed much to preventing mortality during the shock phase. Using the etiologic categorization described by MacLean,[9] the primary cause of shock in a burn patient is hypovolemia. All patients with major thermal injuries and many with more minor injuries and concomitant injuries or diseases need to be evaluated for and possibly treated for hypovolemia. In all such patients, a component of cardiogenic shock must be recognized and treated. Fluid therapy is even more critical for victims of smoke inhalation therapy, since overload and subsequent development of a cardiogenic shock component are easily precipitated.

Resuscitation monitoring

If a patient has hypovolemia, adequate fluid therapy is essential. In the burn patient capillary permeability and thus fluid loss persist for up to 72 hours. Whereas patients with hypovolemic shock from blood loss are treated by stopping hemorrhage followed by volume replacement, in the burn patient it is not possible to stop, diminish, or completely replace the loss. During this initial period the goal is to provide enough volume for adequate perfusion of the vital organs and no more. Since it is not completely possible to determine this amount, the duration of this phase, or the adverse effect of other organs (e.g., the heart and kidneys), careful monitoring and evaluating the effects of fluid therapy are critical.[4]

Nine critical measurements that should be monitored in the patient with a major thermal injury are listed in the box below.

Measurements to be monitored in thermal injury

1. Arterial blood pressure
2. Pulse rate, rhythm, and, by calculation, the rate-pressure product
3. Central venous pressure (CVP) and/or pulmonary capillary wedge pressure (PCWP)
4. Cardiac output and, by calculation,
   a. Cardiac index
   b. Stroke index
   c. Systemic vascular resistance
   d. Left-ventricular stroke index
   e. Right-ventricular stroke index
   f. Pulmonary vascular resistance
   g. Contractility estimation by plotting left-ventricular end-diastolic pressure against cardiac output
5. Arterial blood Po_2, Pco_2, pH, and, by derivation or secondary measurement,
   a. Arterial oxygen content
   b. Mixed venous O_2 tension
   c. Physiologic shunt
   d. Arteriovenous oxygen content difference
6. Hemoglobin/hematocrit concentration
7. Urine flow and, by secondary measurement,
   a. Specific gravity
   b. Urine to plasma creatinine concentration ratio
   c. Urine sodium concentration
8. Mental state
9. Electrolyte concentrations in plasma

Vital signs. Vital signs such as pulse and blood pressure can only be general indications of the level of hypovolemia and the need for fluid replacement. A degree of tachycardia is common, and blood pressure may not reflect perfusion. Trends are important when viewed in perspective with organs such as the kidneys that are dependent on adequate perfusion or blood flow.

Renal output. Renal output does reflect perfusion of the kidneys, which usually also reflects perfusion of other vital organs. This may be misleading in the cases of high-output renal failure, diabetes, and renal disease. These limitations and the dangers inherent in overloading the system are discussed later in this chapter.

Central venous pressure. Measurement of CVP has been especially useful in managing hypovolemia in the young. However, in older patients and those with known cardiopulmonary insufficiency, measurement of PCWP with a Swan-Ganz catheter is essential. When the left-ventricular ejection fraction drops below 40%, the correlation between right-atrial pressure measured by CVP and PCWP is poor. Although shock always has some degree of cardiac dysfunction because of acidosis, decreased oxygen perfusion, or possibly a specific cardiac depressant factor, CVP is most readily available, relatively easy to insert, and has minimal complications. It should be used before a Swan-Ganz catheter in most cases.

Swan-Ganz catheter. The pulmonary artery pressure (PAP) is monitored by use of a Swan-Ganz catheter. PAP is low immediately following injury. During resuscitation 25 to 40 torr correlates with pulmonary vascular resistance and interstitial pulmonary fluid. Normal pulmonary artery end-diastolic pressure, 10 to 20 torr, also correlates with the left-atrial pressure and thus left-ventricular function; higher levels indicate overload or cardiogenic pathology. PAP may be normal even with severe smoke inhalation. Although similar to the results of CVP, PAP is more sensitive to changes in blood volume, cardiac function, and smoke-induced pulmonary edema.[7]

Laboratory studies. Laboratory studies such as hematocrit, hemoglobin, osmotic pressure, pH, blood gases, and electrolytes are all invaluable both as baselines and as indications of the effectiveness of resuscitation efforts. No one test, however, can be viewed as the key. In fact at this time little can be done about hemoconcentration, abnormal osmotic pressure, or hypoproteinemia, other than to observe for trends.

Colloid vs. crystalloid

Indications. A continuing controversy surrounds the use of colloid vs. crystalloid solutions in the treatment of hypovolemic shock. This is true not only for burn shock, but also for hemorrhagic shock and even to some extent cardiogenic shock. Therefore it is important to review the pros and cons of each of these solutions and to be able to recognize and treat the side effects inherent with any resuscitative efforts using these.[2-4,10,11]

Pathophysiologic basis. In a study of 53 extensively burned patients reported by Yoshioka and associates[15] in 1980, the total amount of infusion required to resuscitate the patient in the initial hypovolemic phase was least in the group using hypertonic saline solution, whereas total sodium intake was greatest in the lactated Ringer's solution group. The respiratory index in the hypotonic lactated saline solution group was slightly more elevated than normal, but not significantly. Cardiac output initially decreased in all three groups, but a hyperdynamic state with simultaneous increase in the respiratory index occurred rapidly in the lactated Ringer's group and within 5 to 7 days in the other groups. The Ringer's lactate group and the colloid-plus Ringer's lactate groups revealed no differences in arteriovenous oxygen content.

In 1984 Demling, Kramer, and Harms[5] and Demling and associates[6] reported that burn-induced hypoproteinemia plays a major role in the edema process in nonburn tissues and is corrected by restoration of plasma proteins. Edema in burn tissue does not appear to be related to this process.

In a study by Goodwin and associates[8] in 1983, 79 patients received lactated Ringer's solution or 2.5% albumin-lactated Ringer's solution. Crystalloid-treated patients required more resuscitation than those receiving colloid solution (3.81 vs. 2.98 ml per kilogram of body weight per percent body surface burn, $p < 0.01$). Cardiac index was lower 12 to 24 hours postburn in the crystalloid group, but this difference between treatment groups disappeared 48 hours postburn. Ejection fractions were normal throughout the entire study, whereas the mean rate of internal circumferential fiber shortening (V cf) was supranormal and equal in the two resuscitation groups.

In the second phase of the study (50 patients) extravascular lung water (EVLW) and cardiac index were measured by a standard rebreathing technique during the first week postburn. Lung water remained unchanged in the crystalloid-treated patients but progressively increased in the colloid-treated patients during the 7-day study. Cardiac index increased progressively and identically in both treatment groups. These data refute the existence of myocardial depression during postburn resuscitation and document hypercontractile left-ventricular performance. The addition of colloid to crystalloid resuscitation fluid produces no long-lasting benefit and promotes accumulation of lung water when edema fluid is being reabsorbed from the burn wound.

In 1980 Tranbaugh and associates[14] noted that respiratory failure after thermal injury is common. They used the thermal, green-dye, double-indicator dilution measurement of EVLW to follow daily lung water changes in seven severely burned adult patients resuscitated only with crystalloid solution. They had an average weight gain of 21.3 kg or 30% 2 to 3 days after admission. The authors concluded that massive crystalloid resuscitation maintains pulmonary arterial wedge pressure (PAWP) below 15 torr but does not cause an increase in EVLW during the first 4 days after thermal injury. EVLW actually decreased slightly in all patients despite marked weight gain, hypoproteinemia, and a negative plasma colloid osmotic pressure (PCOP)-PAWP gradient. Three patients had severe inhalation injury and normal

EVLW for the first 4 postburn days. Therefore it appeared that significant interstitial edema did not result from inhalation injury and that thermal injury did not cause an early increase in pulmonary capillary permeability. The occurrence of sepsis resulted in a rapid accumulation of lung water.

To understand the insensitivity of lung water to hemodilution following crystalloid resuscitation, it is necessary to examine Starling's hypothesis. Demling, Kramer, and Harms[5] demonstrated the importance of the osmotic gradient compensation in crystalloid-resuscitated sheep with a 40% body surface burn. They found that lowered PCOP was offset by a proportional lowering of pulmonary lymph osmotic pressure, so that after 48 hours there was no evidence of interstitial fluid accumulation. Starling's hypothesis makes sense only if a normal situation exists. It does not apply when the capillary barrier is abnormal such as with a major thermal injury. In these cases Starling's hypothesis can only be used approximately.

Zarins and colleagues[16] plasmapheresed baboons until PCOP was reduced by 76% of its initial value. A negative PCOP-PAWP gradient resulted, marked peripheral edema and ascites developed, and pulmonary edema did not occur as expected. Pulmonary lymph flow increased sevenfold and pulmonary lymph osmotic pressure decreased 11 torr, protecting the lung from edema formation.

If colloid is to be used, it should be in the form of albumin. Plasma should never be used merely for its oncotic properties. Whether to use a 5% or a 25% albumin depends on the clinical problem. For example, 25% concentration would be best for the immediate postcapillary leak phase early in the course of treatment.

Transfusions. Red blood cell transfusions should only be given when specifically indicated by blood loss such as nonburn wound bleeding or early or late excision. The form of replacement is not different from other medical or surgical situations; i.e., there is no absolute requirement for whole blood. Packed red blood cells (RBCs) will provide the same oxygen support as the equivalent number of RBCs in whole blood. Depending on the clinical situation, it may not be necessary to make up the difference in volume and constituents, or it may be made up by providing the appropriate component.

The need for rapid volume replacement may have different causes at different times during the postburn period. These differences may also influence the type of replacement. Shock because of gram-negative sepsis later in the postburn period and interstitial fluid loss because of capillary insufficiency in the immediate burn period may be treated with crystalloid, but colloid may be more appropriate during the second 24 hours. If rapid volume replacement is necessary at a time when RBC volume is already marginal or low, RBCs may need to be part of the rapid volume replacement. Now that most packed RBCs are suspended in a saline base rather than plasma, flow rates may be very rapid.

To prevent or to identify and treat transfusion reactions, the same precautions and measures should be taken with burn patients as with general patients, but reactions may be more difficult to detect in the septic or febrile patient. In addition, hives may not be detectable in patients with extensive burns. Although prevention of allergic reactions by premedication with antihistamines is acceptable with transfusions of RBCs and components, most physicians are reluctant to use any type of antipyretics with RBCs. Elective transfusions should be given when possible while patients are afebrile or at least not on a rising fever curve, or within 3 to 4 hours of a dose of antipyretics.

In red blood transfusions, microaggregates have been associated with depletion of fibronectin in blood recipients and polymorphonuclear (PMN) dysfunction in burn patients. It is possible to avoid both leukocyte-mediated febrile transfusion reactions and the microaggregate-mediated fibronectin depletion in most instances by the use of microaggregate filters when the blood is administered, or by using frozen or washed blood. The latter modality has the advantage of virtually eliminating allergic transfusion reactions. In view of the difficulty in diagnosing febrile and allergic reactions in burn patients and the potential severe outcome of an allergic reaction, the additional cost of frozen or washed cells or ultrafiltration can be justified in the clinical milieu.

The best prevention for transfusion complications is to avoid unnecessary transfusions. Identification of reactions requires meticulous observation for hypotension, chest pain, pain along the course of the receiving vein, rash, wheezing, dyspnea, and pulmonary edema. Treatment consists of immediate termination of the transfusion and treatment of hemolysis or pulmonary edema. Fever not caused by hemolysis may be treated with antipyretics, but usually ceases when the transfusion is stopped. Fever accompanying transfusions of RBCs, platelets, plasma, and cryoprecipitates should lead to Gram stain and culture of the transfusion apparatus, the donor blood, and the patient's blood. The suspect RBCs should be drawn in citrate and in a clotting tube immediately after the transfusion is stopped. A clotted specimen should be acquired approximately 6 hours later, and urine specimens (not pooled but examined for hemoglobinuria as passed) for several hours following the incident.

Amount and rate determination

Pathophysiology. The goal of fluid therapy is to provide enough volume to maintain vital functions. Total replacement is not possible until the capillary permeability in the burn wound and in the lungs has started to diminish or has ceased.

Formulas. Formulas are a necessary double-edged sword. Based on an approximate correlation between the estimated amount and rate of fluid lost per weight and percent total BSA burned, they are intended as general beginning guidelines only. If the exact amount of fluid given during the resuscitation phase closely approximates the amount of fluid calculated in the beginning using any of the formulas, it is coincidental! Although resuscitation fluid catch-up may be indicated, it is limited by the ability of the body to handle the load, regardless of the calculated or even real

Corollaries of burn fluid management

1. The basic cause of the shock is hypovolemia resulting from capillary and systemic permeability in the burn wound.
2. There is also a secondary degree of increased capillary permeability in the lung.
3. The leakage in the burn wound will start to repair itself in 24 to 48 hours, regardless of the treatment, and will be complete in about 72 to 96 hours.
4. Nothing specific can be done to alter the capillary permeability or its duration at present.
5. The amount of leakage and subsequent edema can be lessened by reduction in fluid given.
6. Reduction in fluids may result in decreased perfusion of vital organs such as the brain, heart, kidneys, and liver.
7. During this initial phase the goal is to provide enough fluid for adequate perfusion of these vital organs and no more.
8. Excess fluid will result in an unnecessary increase in tissue edema, interstitial pulmonary edema, and even cardiogenic shock with heart failure and pulmonary edema, which may be directly or indirectly fatal but at the very least will contribute significantly to morbidity.
9. The capillaries regain their function gradually, starting with the larger molecules, i.e., protein, then the ions and water.
10. There is always a degree of acidosis as a result of the shock, poor tissue perfusion, and anaerobic metabolism.
11. The main initial concerns in fluid management are volume and provision of a buffer for the acidosis.
12. Larger molecules are seldom needed during the early phase or at least until the capillaries can retain them, approximately 24 to 36 hours.
13. Blood, red cells, calcium, and other components are rarely needed unless there is another site of loss besides the burn.
14. The renal output is an excellent method for assessing perfusion of other vital organs unless the patient is a diabetic, develops high output renal failure, has previous renal disease, or has acute renal failure.
15. Increased volume replacement beyond that required for minimal perfusion will not prevent renal shutdown.
16. Fluid should never be given solely on the basis of a "low" central venous pressure.
17. A continuously rising CVP is primarily useful in monitoring the ability of the heart to handle the fluid load by measuring the pressure in the right atrium and thus indicating present or impending cardiac failure.
18. Conversely, an elevated CVP, i.e., > 16 torr, may not reflect the left ventricular filling pressure in the presence of cardiac dysfunction, especially that caused by preexisting cardiac disease. In these cases the CVP may be low with a high wedge or the CVP may be high with a low wedge (i.e., < 8).
19. Cardiac failure can occur, mainly in patients with cardiac pathology, in the presence of hypovolemic shock and must be specifically treated.
20. Enthusiastic and unwatched fluid replacement can rapidly put a patient in heart failure.
21. A Foley catheter is obligatory in the management of a major burn. Urinary tract infection may be inevitable, but the risk is considered acceptable.
22. Instead of compensating for variability and maintenance of perfusion with changes in volume, hypertonic sodium solution can be used. This will result in less infused volume during the early shock phase, but as yet it has not been shown to alter morbidity or mortality. It is also considerably more difficult to monitor the essential parameters with the use of hypertonic sodium than with Ringer's lactate; therefore it is not generally recommended unless the personnel and facility are proficient in its use.

Continued.

Corollaries of burn fluid management—cont'd

23. Following the resuscitation phase in a major burn injury, the primary cause of edema into nonburned tissue is hypoproteinemia. This is not a factor in burned tissue during the immediate postburn period, even though the hypoproteinemia can occur within the first few hours. Infusion of large amounts of colloid, i.e., plasma, during this period is therefore of little value.

---

need. As listed in the box on pp. 97 and 98, a number of corollaries should be adhered to in managing fluid therapy in the patient with a major thermal injury.

The Evans, Brooke, and Parkland formulas are commonly used in the determination of amounts of fluid required.

Evans. The Evans formula, introduced in 1952, was one of the first that correlated the amount of fluid required[1,12] with both the body weight and the percent of total BSA burned. In addition, by dividing the amount into a gradually decreasing rate, it reflected the gradual lessening of the capillary permeability.

> First 12 hours: 2 ml/kg/% BSA
> Second 12 hours: 1 ml/kg/% BSA
> Second 24 hours: 1 ml/kg/% BSA

Brooke. In contrast to the Evans formula, the Brooke formula specifies the type of fluid given and adds an amount for insensible water loss.

> Colloids: 0.5 ml/%BSA/kg
> Lactated Ringer's solution: 1.5 ml/%BSA/kg
> Water requirement (D_5W):   2000 ml for adults, children correspondingly less

The second 24-hour period requirements for the colloids and lactated Ringer's solution are one half those for the initial 24 hours.

In calculating the fluid requirements, the maximum allowed is that for a 50% total BSA burn and includes second- and third-degree areas.

Parkland. The Parkland formula is a derivation of one designed by Moyer in which resuscitation is only with lactated Ringer's solution. For initial guidance, 4 ml/kg with a urine output of 30 to 70 ml/hour is given. Thereafter the amount of fluid is determined by monitoring the patient.

According to Baxter,[1] using the Parkland formula,[13] patients with an inhalation injury required 37% additional fluid over the calculations to maintain output. This is nearly 4 L of additional Ringer's lactate during the first 24 hours.

Oral fluids

Indications for oral fluids. Generally, all patients with a major thermal injury should be given nothing by mouth under ordinary circumstances. If it appears that the patient can tolerate oral fluid, it must be appreciated that ileus may develop as late as several hours following any injury. In either case it is hazardous to depend on any oral fluid for resuscitation.

Nasogastric suction. Nasogastric suction should be used on specific indication, i.e., nausea and vomiting or abdominal distention that is uncomfortable or interferes with coughing and ventilation.

Use of antacids and histamine receptor antagonists. Histamine receptor antagonists (e.g., cimetidine) should be used if there is a history of peptic ulcer disease. The popular use of antacids is probably not the cause of the marked reduction in the occurrence of Curling's ulcer, nor is the use of histamine receptor antagonists. Since there are little or no side effects with either treatment, they can be used as warranted.

Nutritional evaluation and support

There is some indication that the early use of hyperalimentation, either parenterally or orally, is of value in healing. As a practical matter, it is difficult to institute during the acute resuscitation phase. The patient should be evaluated and started on therapy as soon as the shock phase has subsided and even during the diuresis phase. Every patient with a major thermal injury, and many of those with a minor one, should receive some level of nutritional support.

PROBLEMS WITH FLUID THERAPY

A number of clinical problems are frequently encountered and somewhat unique to the treatment of the thermally injured patient. They fall into several categories such as those related to fluid therapy or those unique to the burn wound (e.g., constriction of the thoracic cage or of an extremity caused by the swelling of a circumferential burn, hypertension, development of Curling's ulcer, hypothermia, or idiopathic diabetes).

The approach to both the recognition and treatment of these problems depends not only on a knowledge of critical care pathophysiology, but most important and often lacking, a thorough understanding of the pathophysiology of the burn injury and the often adverse effects of therapy. Considering the nexus of these dynamic events, the presentation is most readily resolved with the aid of a checklist format.

Response to fluid challenge

The use of a fluid challenge can often serve as a reliable diagnostic indication as to whether a problem (specifically, hypovolemic or cardiogenic shock) is being

Table 6-1. The 5-2 rule

For a CVP*	Infuse	Over
CVP < 8	200 ml	10 minutes
14 > CVP > 8	100 ml	10 minutes
CVP > 14	50 ml	10 minutes

*Pressures are in centimeters of H_2O.

Table 6-2. The 7-3 rule

For a wedge*	Infuse	Over
Wedge < 12	200 ml	10 minutes
16 > Wedge > 12	100 ml	10 minutes
Wedge > 16	50 ml	10 minutes

*Pressures are in torr.

inadequately treated. Furthermore, since these entities commonly occur in combinations, each with varying impact, the infusion challenge can provide valuable guidelines in planning the treatment. The CVP 5-2 rule and the pulmonary wedge pressure obtained with a Swan-Ganz catheter or the wedge 7-3 rule are frequently used in a challenge test.

CVP 5-2 rule. Table 6-1 illustrates the application of the CVP 5-2 rule. If the CVP rises more than 5 cm, the fluid challenge is stopped. If the CVP rises less than 2 cm in response to the infusion, a repeat challenge should be administered.

If the CVP rises 2 to 5 cm as a result of the challenge, the patient should be observed for 10 minutes; if the CVP remains 2 to 5 cm above baseline, no further challenges are given. If the CVP has fallen to within 2 cm of the baseline, the challenge is repeated.

7-3 rule. If the wedge pressure rises more than 7 mm in response to the infusion, a repeat challenge should be administered.

If the wedge rises 3 to 7 mm as a result of the infusion, the patient should be observed for 10 minutes. If the wedge remains 3 to 7 mm above baseline, no further challenges are given. If the wedge has fallen to within 3 mm of baseline, the challenge is repeated. These guidelines are shown in Table 6-2.

Hypovolemia

Hypovolemia is usually caused by inadequate evaluation of the depth and extent of the burn wound, delay in starting fluid replacement therapy, or reluctance to give the often large amounts of fluid required for fear of overload and inducing congestive heart failure. Use of inadequate access lines and failure to appreciate other losses can also contribute to this condition. Failure to promptly correct the hypovolemia will result in prolongation of the shock status, renal shutdown, and finally death. Rapid catch-up can also result in fluid overload and heart failure, thereby starting an ominous cycle of events. The signs and treatment of hypovolemia are as follows:

1. Signs
   a. Decreased urinary output
   b. Fall in blood pressure
   c. Low CVP
   d. Rising BUN
2. Treatment
   a. Increased amount of crystalloid
   b. Increased rate of administration
   c. Possible use of osmotic diuretic if concerned about renal shutdown. (A response to furosemide may be misleading, since it has been shown to increase urine output in the presence of hypovolemia. Its use still may be valuable, but the results must be interpreted with caution or awareness.)

Anemia

Anemia is not common during the immediate postburn period unless there is a preexisting bleeding disease or reasons other than thermal injury for the blood loss. Bleeding from Curling's ulcer has become rare during the past few years, but it can occur as early as 1 day postburn. In a major burn patient it is much more common to find anemia following resuscitation caused by dilution; after the diuresis phase anemia is caused by repeated phlebotomy, debridement, and depression of the bone marrow. This occurs approximately at the fifth to seventh day postburn. The causes, diagnoses, and treatment of anemia are as follows:

1. Causes
   a. Internal bleeding
   b. Inadequate blood replacement
   c. Overwhelming hemolysis, usually septic in origin
   d. Fat emboli
2. Diagnosis
   a. Sudden fall in hematocrit
   b. Signs and symptoms of hypovolemia
3. Treatment
   a. Blood transfusion as indicated
   b. Treatment of the cause of the anemia

Overload syndrome

Overload syndrome is not uncommon and usually results from a failure to appreciate the difference between hypovolemic shock resulting from hemorrhage and that caused by the increased capillary permeability found in burn shock. In the former, once the bleeding is controlled, the volume can be replaced as rapidly as the cardiopulmonary system can handle the load. In the latter case, however, the loss through the capillary walls will only diminish as the capillaries regain their function; and, until that time (approximately 2 to 3 days), attempts to completely correct the loss will only result in occurrence of an overload syndrome. The tendencies (1) to retrospectively replace the urine output without regard to the diuretic phase, or (2) to administer fluid on the basis of a low or normal CVP in order to better restore intravascular fluid volume are frequent examples of a lack of appreciation of thermal injury pathophysiology. Suggestions for the diagnosis and treatment of overload syndrome are listed in the box below.

Congestive heart failure

Even with a so-called normal heart, there is some degree of cardiogenic or congestive heart failure in every patient with a major thermal injury during some phase of resuscitation. For example, gradually increasing CVP readings are common to all major resuscitation efforts. This is easily understandable even without the demonstration of the production of a thermal myocardial depressant factor, which some have advocated, but simply because of decreased perfusion of oxygen with

---

Diagnosis and treatment of overload syndrome

1. Diagnosis
   a. Rales
   b. Pulmonary edema on x-ray film
   c. Enlarged liver
   d. Cerebral edema
   e. Peripheral edema unrelated to the burn site
   f. Increased urine output and decreased specific gravity
   g. Elevated CVP
   h. Administration of fluid greatly in excess of calculated requirements
   i. Electrocardiographic evidence of left ventricular strain
2. Treatment
   a. Reduce input, especially sodium
   b. Lasix (furosemide)
   c. Digitalize: Digoxin 0.03-0.05 mg/kg IM or IV over 24 hours in divided doses

lowered availability of adequate tissue perfusion and acidosis secondary to all types of shock. In a patient with some cardiovascular disease, cardiac failure is even more likely to occur.

The goal during resuscitation is not only prevention of inadequate perfusion by careful monitoring and adjustment of the fluid therapy, but prompt treatment. In this regard, many recommend prophylactic digitalization under the concept that the myocardium is not normal in a patient with major injury and shock and that slower digitalization is more controllable. On the other hand, today's monitoring techniques, together with present pharmaceuticals, permit a more rapid and specific correction of deficits than were formerly possible.

A practical compromise depends on the availability of monitoring equipment and a cardiologist familiar with critical care and thermal injury patients, in which case routine digitalization is not recommended.

As indicated, the CVP is most sensitive to impending cardiac failure, and a rising CVP indicates this event. Although the first treatment is usually to reduce fluid intake, it may not be possible to do this and yet maintain urine output. Therefore the next approach is to treat the cardiogenic component with specific cardiotropic agents and to try diuretic therapy. If this is not successful, there may be no choice but to reduce fluid intake. Occasionally, changing to colloid at this point may be helpful in reducing volume yet maintaining osmotic pressure. In a patient with a massive thermal injury, these events often precede total vascular collapse and death.

Digitalization regimen for congestive heart failure and selected large burns is as follows:
1. Rapid digitalization:
   ½ total digitalizing dose stat IM or IV; ¼ at 6-hour intervals
2. Routine digitalization:
   ¼ digitalizing dose divided into quarterly doses and given at 6-hour intervals
3. Maintenance dosage:
   ¼ of digitalizing dose divided into two equal doses and given at 12-hour intervals IM or PO

Water intoxication/hypoelectrolytemia

The cause of this phenomenon is closely related to that previously described for water intoxication. The difference is that in the case of hypoelectrolytemia, fluid therapy has been primarily with a dextrose in water solution as opposed to a balanced and buffered crystalloid solution such as Ringer's lactate. The clinical findings are more dramatic and not necessarily related to congestive heart failure. The diagnosis and treatment of hypoelectrolytemia is listed in the box on p. 104.

Hypoelectrolytemia can also occur with high output renal failure. In these cases, the distal renal tubules fail to reabsorb the electrolytes, particularly sodium, resulting in severe imbalances.

Diagnosis and treatment of hypoelectrolytemia

1. Diagnosis
   a. Mental confusion proceeding to convulsions
   b. Sodium below 130 mEq/L
   c. Chloride below 80 mEq/L
   d. Decreased serum osmolarity
   e. Decreased specific gravity
   f. Administration of water (usually D_5W) in excess of calculated requirements
   g. Often confused clinically with acute gram-negative sepsis
2. Treatment
   a. Restrict free water
   b. Hypertonic NaCl:
   mEq NaCl = body weight (kg) $\times$ 0.6 $\times$ 5 (or body weight times the % body distribution
          of Na times the usual correction factor; can be plus or minus, depending
          on the deficit of Na in the body)
          3% NaCl = 0.5 mEq/ml
          5% NaCl = 0.85 mEq/ml
   c. Reduce IV input to minimum for 6 to 12 hours

Acidosis

Acidosis, often severe, is found to some degree in all shock patients. It is most apparent in burn patients treated only with saline solution rather than with a balanced and buffered salt solution, as was commonly the practice years ago. This event can also be complicated by respiratory acidosis, which can further shift the oxygen dissociation curve and reduce tissue perfusion. What is found, clinically, is a combination of these factors and corrections, which at first can be treated by buffering with intravenous sodium bicarbonate but which will eventually require a broad correction of the pathophysiology. Immediate diagnosis and treatment are mandatory if the patient is to survive.

Guidelines for the diagnosis and treatment of acidosis are as follows:

1. Diagnosis
   a. Rapid deep respirations
   b. Urine pH below 5.5
   c. Blood pH below 7.35
   d. pCO_2 elevated in respiratory acidosis
   e. CO_2 combining power decreased in metabolic acidosis
2. Treatment
   a. Adjustment of ventilatory support equipment
   b. IV sodium bicarbonate

Table 6-3. ECG changes in hyperkalemia

Serum potassium (mEq/L)	ECG
6-7	Tall, peaked T-waves
8	P-waves may disappear or be mixed into QRS
10	Wide, aberrant QRS
11	Biphasic deflections
12	Ventricular fibrillation

Diagnosis and treatment of hyperkalemia

1. Diagnosis
   a. Possible falsely elevated potassium level caused by hemolysis of blood specimen
   b. Usually accompanied by acute renal failure
   c. Acidosis
   d. Excessive administration of potassium
   e. Adrenal cortical insufficiency
2. Treatment
   a. For serum potassium, 7 mEq/L:
      1. Calcium gluconate, 0.5 ml/kg 10% solution over 2 to 4 minutes
      2. Sodium bicarbonate, 2.5 mEq/kg (3 ml/kg) of a 7.5% $NaHCO_3$ solution
      3. 25% or 50% glucose, 1 ml/kg with insulin 1 U/5 g of glucose IV
   b. For serum potassium, 5.5 to 7 mEq/L:
      1. Cation exchange resin or Kayexalate—use 10 to 30 g, depending on body weight
      2. Institution of peritoneal dialysis for intractable hyperkalemia

Hyperkalemia

Probably the most common cause of hyperkalemia (serum potassium < 5.5 mEq/L) in the first few postburn days, with the exception of preexisting disease, is the administration of added potassium in the resuscitation fluid. The amount of potassium in Ringer's lactate is not critical in this regard and is promptly excreted in the urine. Depending on the amount of burn tissue destruction, additional potassium will be absorbed, and there will usually be a modest increase in serum potassium levels from this alone. The most important aspect of this is to be aware that a rapidly dropping serum potassium level may be found once diuresis occurs.

Table 6-3 lists the ECG changes found at various levels of serum potassium. Specific diagnostic and treatment parameters are listed in the box above.

Hyponatremia

The cause of hyponatremia in the early postburn period is usually simple overload, but it also can be high output renal failure. This latter event, in which the physician can be misled by a good urine volume into believing that the resuscitation is going well can be a difficult problem. It is most readily diagnosed by frequent urine tests which note a specific gravity approaching 1.01, together with urine electrolyte determination and serum analysis.

Hypernatremia

Hypernatremia can occur insidiously as a result of inadequate water replacement, failure to appreciate a large insensible fluid loss, and the complacency engendered by a slightly elevated serum sodium level. The onset usually occurs after the acute resuscitation effort has succeeded. The continuously rising sodium levels are thought to be the result of proper fluid management, and the report just before the acute manifestations of hypernatremia are overlooked as a slightly high laboratory result that day. Hypernatremia is manifested by confusion, hypotension, and oliguria. The diagnosis is commonly interpreted as gram-negative sepsis. Although diagnosis may also be valid, the rapid administration (i.e., as much as 1 L/hour or as the cardiovascular system permits) will result in a rapid improvement, which of course is usually not seen that quickly in the treatment of acute septic shock. The total amount of water necessary to correct the condition will vary markedly, but as much as 5 or more liters of additional fluid in a 24-hour period would not be unusual.

Prerenal oliguria

Prerenal oliguria can occur in the thermally injured patient as a result of hypovolemia, inadequate resuscitation, dehydration either from gastrointestinal losses or evaporative losses, hemorrhage, or excessive diuretics. The treatment depends first on recognition of the cause and then on the specific correction of the problem.

Renal oliguria

Acute tubular necrosis (ATN). ATN is a possibility, and the best prevention is careful fluid management. If it occurs, renal dialysis should be considered. Fortunately, this is rarely required during the immediate postburn period while the patient is being stabilized, unless there is preexisting renal disease.

Myoglobinuria or hemoglobinuria. The finding of hemoglobinuria or myoglobinuria can be ominous. It usually indicates a very severe burn extending to the muscle

Table 6-4. Diagnostic comparison of oliguria and ATN

	Diagnostic oliguria	ATN
Urine specific gravity	1.015	1.01
Radio-urine (osmol/plasma)	500	320
Urine sodium (mEq/L)	20, usually 10	20, usually 40
Urea (urine/plasma)	15:1	10:1
Creatinine (urine/plasma)	15:1	10:1

and deep tissues, which in itself usually precludes survival. In addition, resuscitation is difficult, and often the tendency is to increase fluid intake with the primary goal of diluting the urine and preventing renal shutdown. Unfortunately, this doesn't work and only tends to overload the patient. If the patient survives the first few days, in all likelihood renal dialysis will be required.

Drugs. Some drugs (e.g., gentamicin or amphotericin) required during the immediate postburn period are excreted by the kidneys and should be avoided if possible. If a drug (e.g., gentamicin) is needed for extensive sepsis by day 5 to 7, the dosage needs to be calculated carefully, levels obtained if possible, and prolonged retention anticipated.

Diagnostic tests for oliguria. A diagnostic comparison between oliguria and ATN is shown in Table 6-4. In addition, the following infusion or water-load tests can be of value.

1. Water-load test:
   D_5W, 300 ml/m² over 30 minutes; must be done with constant CVP monitoring
2. Mannitol infusion test:
   0.2 g/kg over 5 to 10 minutes (20% solution)
3. Diuretic challenge:
   Furosemide (Lasix)—in adults, 20 to 80 mg; in children, 2 mg/kg; or ethacrynic acid (Edecrin)—1 mg/kg

High-output renal failure

This complication is diagnosed by high urine output of low specific gravity. Its occurrence generally is accompanied by an elevated urinary sodium loss that makes the further rate and amount of urine output unreliable for management monitoring. The treatment is fluid restriction and the judicious use of hypertonic sodium chloride solution. This therapy should be followed closely by frequent testing of both the urine and serum electrolytes.

Diabetes mellitus or insipidus

Pseudodiabetes has been reported to occur in approximately 1% of major burn patients. It is characteristically diagnosed by inordinate glycosuria, high renal output, and resistant acidosis. The treatment is IV insulin in often large amounts and as needed. It is termed "pseudo" because no diabetes is evident following recovery.

REFERENCES

1. Baxter, CR: Guidelines for fluid therapy, J Trauma 21:687, 1981.
2. Burke, JF: Resuscitative fluid composition, J Trauma 21:692, 1981.
3. Caldwell, FT: Hypertonic saline, J Trauma 21:693, 1981.
4. Civetta, JM: Intensive care therapeutics, New York, 1980, Appleton-Century-Crofts.
5. Demling, RH, Kramer, G, and Harms, B: Role of thermal injury-induced hypoproteinemia on fluid flux and protein permeability in burned and nonburned tissue, Surgery 95:136, 1984.
6. Demling, RH, et al: Effect of burn induced hypoproteinemia on pulmonary transvascular fluid filtration rate, Surgery 85:339, 1979.
7. German, JC, Allyn, PA, and Bartlett, RH: Pulmonary artery pressure monitoring in acute burn management, Arch Surg 106:788, 1973.
8. Goodwin, CW, et al: Randomized trial of efficacy of crystalloid and colloid resuscitation on hemodynamic response and lung water following thermal injury, Ann Surg 197:520, 1983.
9. MacLean, LD: A century of progress, Ann Surg 201:407, 1985.
10. Monafo, WW: The role of albumin in burn resuscitation, J Trauma 21:694, 1981.
11. Monafo, WW, Halverson, JD, and Schectman, K: The role of concentrated sodium solutions in the resuscitation of patients with severe burns, Surgery 95:129, 1984.
12. Pruitt, BA, Jr: Fluid resuscitation for extensively burned patients, J Trauma 21:690, 1981.
13. Scheulin, JJ, and Munster, AM: The Parkland formula in patients with burns and inhalation injury, J Trauma 22:869, 1982.
14. Tranbaugh, RF, et al: Lung water changes after thermal injury: the effects of crystalloid resuscitation and sepsis, Ann Surg 192:479, 1980.
15. Yoshioka, T, et al: Effect of intravenously administered fluid on hemodynamic change and respiratory function in extensive thermal injury, Surg Gynecol Obstet 151:503, 1980.
16. Zarins, CK, et al: Lymph and pulmonary response to isobaric reduction in plasma oncotic pressure in baboons, Circ Res 43:925, 1978.

7 Respiratory Care

INJURY TO THE RESPIRATORY SYSTEM

Direct or indirect injury to the respiratory system has emerged as the major cause of death in patients with thermal injury. Such injury may take the form of a direct injury caused by inhalation of the products of combustion, or an indirect injury from the effects of shock or products produced in the burn wound, or a combination of adverse effects on the lung's bacterial defense mechanisms.[4]

Application of the many advances in critical medicine have done much to treat the sequelae of these problems, particularly airway obstruction, pulmonary insufficiency, and edema. There has been little improvement in treating those patients who develop acute respiratory distress syndrome (ARDS) or profound loss of bacterial defense mechanisms. Yet some advances have been made in reducing the incidence of ARDS, especially in patients with smaller burns, and in indirectly enhancing the body's defense with better nutritional support, earlier wound closure, and prevention of burn wound sepsis.[9]

The objective of respiratory care can be defined as the provision of adequate respiration through ventilation with either the least effect on, or, if possible, some enhancement of the cardiopulmonary hemodynamics, and with the least adverse effect on the host defense mechanisms.

A direct thermal injury to the respiratory tract can result in a massive occlusion of the airway because of either heat or the inhalation of irritating pyrolysates. This occurrence requires prompt recognition and treatment. As discussed on p. 57, tracheostomy is not recommended unless an airway or nasotracheal or endotracheal intubation is impossible because of severe injuries to the maxillofacial area. Early

109

pulmonary insufficiency not relieved by prompt endotracheal intubation and ventilation is usually fatal.

The lung lesions associated with pure, thermal damage to the dermis involve an increase in lung lymph flow and edema formation. During the resuscitation phase these fluid losses, i.e., edema, are usually replaced by crystalloid solutions with no colloid content, so that the patient may be functionally hypoproteinemic and have an elevated metabolic rate with a corresponding increase in cardiac output and, consequently, pulmonary blood flow. This increased perfusion of the pulmonary capillaries may further increase edema formation.

As the lesions progress, a castlike material composed of fibrin can cause partial or complete obstruction of large and small airways, resulting in patches of atelectasis.

An examination of the lung lymph shows an elevated ratio of lymph-to-plasma protein concentration, in contrast to the hydrostatic edema of congestive heart failure. Cardiac output and left atrial pressure are either normal or reduced, indicating a microvascular permeability change.

Following inhalation injury, blood is shunted from ventilated to nonventilated areas of the lung, which compounds the problem of providing adequate ventilation.

Perhaps the most important factor in survival is the marked fall in lung compliance. Changes in lung compliance are associated with a deficiency of surfactant activity; similar findings are reported in patients with ARDS. These changes are attributed to abnormalities in the chemical composition of the lung surfactant phospholipids. Since it appears that surfactant enhances the function of the alveolar macrophages, surfactant deficiency is also related to the high incidence of pulmonary sepsis.

In treatment of inhalation injury, prompt recognition, oxygen administration, airway relief, and intravenous bronchodilators can provide dramatic relief, particularly if the patient has a severe bronchospasm because of an irritant or allergen. In more serious cases, appropriate ventilatory support can be lifesaving.

TYPES OF CARE

Abbreviations used in this section can be found in the box on p. 111. Control of the upper airway is vital.[2] Either nasotracheal or endotracheal intubation is acceptable. Although more difficult to insert and often of smaller diameter, the nasotracheal tube is more comfortable. Ideally the tube should have a soft, alternating pressure cuff that lessens damage to the laryngeal tracheal wall.[7,19]

Many authors have reported the onset of severe, noncardiac pulmonary edema within minutes of intubation. Fluid overload with concomitant hydrostatic edema formation must be carefully avoided. The principle of keeping patients in a slightly underhydrated state has been questioned in recent years, because a fluid requirement is necessary for the patient's other needs, i.e., renal function and maintenance of

---

Abbreviations

CPAP	Continuous positive airway pressure
CPPB	Continuous positive-pressure breathing
Flo$_2$	Forced inspiratory oxygen
I:E ratio	Inspiratory to expiratory time ratio
IMV	Intermittent mandatory ventilation
IPPB	Intermittent positive-pressure breathing
Paco$_2$	Partial pressure of carbon dioxide in alveolar blood
Pao$_2$	Partial pressure of oxygen in arterial blood
PEEP	Positive end-expiratory pressure
Vd	Dead space volume
V̇e	Minute ventilation
Vt	Tidal volume

---

pulmonary capillary wedge pressure for cardiac output. However, if noncardiac pulmonary edema has occurred, positive pressure ventilation can be lifesaving.[1,6,9,11]

Classification of ventilators by function

Three different types of cycling ventilators are commonly available: assistor ventilators, controller ventilators, and intermittent mandatory ventilators.

Assistor ventilators are triggered by the patient and deliver a full volume. They are most effective with a cooperative patient and IPPB during weaning.

Controller ventilators are reset at a certain rate regardless of the patient's ability to trigger the apparatus. This is useful when the patient is unable to make any respiratory effort. The ventilator usually takes control, particularly when the patient is sedated.

IMV is particularly useful in weaning patients by allowing spontaneous breaths, then augmenting these with a prescribed period of forced breaths. IMV is useful for patients who require high levels of positive pressure. At any given pressure the mean intrathoracic pressure is lower, and venous return is affected less with IMV than with conventional mechanical ventilation (CMV).

Classification of ventilators according to phase

Ventilators are also classified by the four phases through which all ventilators pass in each cycle: inspiratory, inspiratory to expiratory, expiratory, and expiratory to inspiratory.

During the inspiratory phase gas is delivered to the lungs. Flow rate, volume,

Table 7-1. Therapeutic objectives of various modes of respiratory care

Type of care	Objective
Oxygen	Provide adequate tissue oxygenation
	Decrease the work of breathing
	Decrease myocardial work
Aerosol therapy	Dry hydrate and retain secretions
	Restore and maintain mucous blanket
	Promote expectoration
	Improve cough effectiveness
	Humidify inspired gas
	Deliver medications
Incentive spirometry	Promote deep breathing
	Improve distribution of ventilation
Endotracheal or nasotracheal intubation	Protect and maintain open airway
	Permit mechanical ventilation
	Prevent aspiration
	Maintain thorough bronchial toilet
Ventilatory support	Provide pulmonary system with mechanical power to maintain physiologic ventilation
	Manipulate the ventilatory pattern and airway pressures for purposes of improving efficiency of ventilation, treatment of hypoxemia
	Regulate Pa_{CO_2}
IPPB	Deliver medications
	Administer drug by IPPB because, when a person has limited breathing ability, this will better distribute the drug
CPAP	Increase alveolar surface area
	Decrease alveolar collapse
	Decrease shunting
	Improve arterial oxygen tension
PEEP	Increase alveolar surface area
	Decrease alveolar collapse
	Decrease shunting
	Improve arterial oxygen tension
IMV	Reduce the amount of time required for mechanical ventilation
	Facilitate weaning of patient from controlled or assisted mechanical ventilation
	Provide a more physiologic way to maintain ventilation
	Allow patient to determine his own $\dot{V}_E$, which in turn sustains a more physiologic Pa_{CO_2}
	Decrease the mean intrathoracic pressure

airway pressure, and composition should be considered. Generators or ventilators can be constant flow, variable flow, pressure, or variable pressure.

In the transition from the inspiratory to the expiratory phase ventilators can be either time-cycled, pressure-cycled, or volume-cycled. Most ventilators in an intensive care unit are volume-cycled ventilators, which will cycle from inspiration to expiration after a preset volume has been delivered. These are equipped with preset safety valves to limit the pressure generated. Leak detection is particularly difficult with this type of ventilator; thus it is necessary to measure exhaled Vts as a control.

Expiratory phase ventilator valves open immediately after full inspiration or after an adjustable waiting period that is called the inspiratory plateau. Often expiration is totally passive, but the ventilator may have options that allow expiratory retard, active expiration, and PEEP. Expiratory retard is a mechanism to slow the rate of exhalation, supposedly to permit a more complete emptying of the lung.

CPAP or PEEP is widely used in this phase.[8,10,12] They are not the same; PEEP means positive pressure only at end expiration (i.e., pressures at any other point may be negative), whereas CPAP is continuous positive pressure throughout the cycle. For example, the patient on IMV who has a varied rate of inspiratory flow during a spontaneous breath may on PEEP produce negative airway pressure on inspiration, whereas the patient on CPAP will always produce positive pressure. The primary objective of positive pressure is to prevent a collapse of the alveoli and small airways. Both PEEP and CPAP can be advantageous but both, used injudiciously, can interfere with venous return to the heart and result in a fall in cardiac output.

The I:E ratio is also a factor that can be controlled. This needs to be individually adjusted in patients with bronchospasm to provide optimal ventilation.

Change from expiratory to inspiratory phase ventilators can be triggered by either the patient or the ventilator. They can be assistor, controller, or intermittent as discussed earlier.

In actual practice commercially available ventilators contain a variable number of controls. They should be used on the basis of physiologic need, familiarity, and reliability.

THERAPEUTIC OBJECTIVES OF VARIOUS TREATMENT MODES

Each of the various modes of therapy available for respiratory care of the thermally injured patient have specific objectives. These are summarized in Table 7-1.

INDICATIONS FOR MECHANICAL VENTILATION

The indications for mechanical ventilation in the burn patient follow:
1. Suspicion of hypoxemia
2. Hypoventilation pH < 7.35 and $Paco_2 > 40$ torr
3. Normal $Paco_2$ and severe metabolic acidosis
4. Respiratory arrest
5. Use of a muscle relaxant or respiratory depressant drug
6. Bradycardia
7. Severe, exhausting dyspnea or tachypnea
8. Increased airway resistance or poor compliance
9. Increased intracranial pressure

10. Inadequate circulation caused by shock
11. Suspected aspiration of gastric contents
12. Increasing $PaCO_2$ or respiratory rate
13. Development of pulmonary edema

Perhaps the most important is a suspicion of hypoxemia. Conditions can change rapidly and insidiously, and, although abundant laboratory tests are now generally available, the inherent time delay in obtaining these data can yield disastrous results.

If intubation is performed, patients should be placed on mechanical ventilation (12 to 15 ml/kg Vt) and CPAP (beginning with 5 cm of H_2O) to maintain small airway patency. Since the primary problem is airway collapse, PEEP should be a major component of ventilatory management.

SPECIFIC INDICATIONS FOR PEEP OR CPAP

Specific indications for either PEEP or CPAP are as follows:
1. Hypoxia
   a. $PaO_2 < 60$ torr on FIO_2 0.5
   b. $PaO_2 < 300$ torr on FIO_2 1
   c. Vd/Vt > 20%
2. Clinical observations
   a. Pulmonary edema
   b. Left-sided heart failure
   c. Pulmonary contusion
   d. Flail chest
   e. Aspiration of gastric contents
   f. Massive fluid resuscitation
   g. Poor parenchymal compliance
   h. Severe bronchospasm
3. Trends
   a. Decreasing PaO_2
   b. Increasing Vd/Vt
4. Other
   a. Bronchospasm

It should be noted that careful monitoring and adjustment are key factors in the successful management of these patients.

Both CPAP and PEEP levels less than 15 cm of H_2O have little effect on the circulation unless the patient is hypovolemic and/or has a markedly reduced cardiac reserve.

The I:E ratio should be adjusted to optimize oxygenation and pulmonary compliance.

If the PaO_2 is less than 70 torr, it is advisable to give Vts of 12 to 15 mL/kg of body weight with a rate of 12 to 16 breaths per minute and an inspiratory-to-expiratory ratio of 1:2. A starting FIO_2 of 0.4 is recommended and can be adjusted to achieve an accepted PaO_2 of 70 to 90 torr.

The therapeutic objectives for ARDS are designed to provide ventilatory support, obviate fatigue, and combine the appropriate Vt, inspiratory pressure, expiratory pressure, and FIO_2 to optimize total oxygenation.

The detrimental effects of PEEP seem to be partially ameliorated by the use of CPAP and IMV. The PEEP-induced decrease in expiratory left ventricular filling is equal to that from CPPB and CPAP; a decrease in inspiratory left ventricular filling is noted only with CPPB.

VENTILATORY ORDERS

Ventilatory orders should be written and reviewed fully and specifically, an example of which is shown in the box below. Usually critical care units have a form on which all of these various items are listed with pertinent monitoring parameters.

WEANING

The most important extubation or weaning advice is not to hurry. Weaning must be planned at time of optimum supervision. At present, tubes have been in place in some patients for up to several months without damage. Removal too soon can result in hypoxemia and pulmonary and cardiac failure. The rush to replace an endotracheal tube with a tracheostomy can lead to both immediate technical and anesthesia complications and the long-term effects of increased pulmonary sepsis and airway stricture. Some of the main considerations in weaning are as follows:

1. Do not hurry!
2. Evaluate for the following:
    a. Secretions
    b. Mental status

Sample ventilatory orders

1. Vt 10-15 cc/kg exhaled, or
   (height in cm × 10) − 800 cc (men)
   (height in cm × 10) − 900 cc (women)
2. Rate 10/minute
3. FIO_2 1
4. PEEP 0-5 cm H_2O
5. I:E::1:2
6. Arterial blood gases (ABGs) in 15 minutes and adjust ventilation and oxygen concentration
7. Suction q2h and prn
8. Nasogastric tube
9. Sedation prn

c. Cardiovascular stability
d. Sepsis
e. Pulmonary edema
f. Ability to maintain airway
g. Compliance
h. Presence of metabolic acidosis

THE RESTLESS PATIENT

Restlessness is a classic sign of hypoxemia. A checklist of problems, shown in the following list, further emphasizes the need to periodically examine the patient:

1. Check vital signs and obtain ABGs
2. Check for airway obstruction in upper airway with kinking, secretions, or exudate or aberrant tube position
3. Check tidal volume with spirometer
4. Check flow in both limbs of ventilatory apparatus for leaks and proper operation
5. Do a chest x-ray examination for atelectasis, hemothorax, or pneumothorax
6. Sedate patient
7. Give analgesics but first check for cause of pain
8. Administer neuromuscular blockers

COMPLICATIONS OF VENTILATORY SUPPORT

A number of complications relate not only to the ventilatory support of the patient, but to the treatment of all of the various interrelated components of the hemodynamic abnormalities found in the burn patient. Complications of three of the most widely used modes of treatment (i.e., intubation, mechanical ventilation, and positive-pressure breathing) are listed in the box on p. 117.

THE PULMONARY HOST DEFENSE MECHANISM[3-5,13-18]

The lung represents the largest surface that the body exposes to the external environment. The total surface area of the alveoli is estimated to be approximately 70 m², or 1 m²/kg of body weight. Like the skin, but with 100 times greater surface area, the lung is constantly threatened by bacterial contamination. Yet the defense mechanisms of the upper and lower airways are so well developed and efficient in protecting the vital gas-exchange area from contamination that the lung usually remains sterile in spite of continuous exposure to a multitude of microorganisms in the air and blood. However, this host defense mechanism is severely taxed in the patient with a major inhalation or thermal injury, and failure can result in fatal sepsis.

Complications related to ventilation

Intubation and airway maintenance

1. Hypoxia
2. Bradycardia
3. Stimulation-agitation, hypertension, and tachycardia
4. Bronchospasm
5. Pulmonary aspiration
6. Esophageal intubation
7. Malpositioning and right upper lobe (RUL) atelectasis
8. Laryngeal damage
9. Tracheal stenosis
10. Infection

Complications of mechanical ventilation

1. Hyperventilation
2. Hypoventilation
3. Barotrauma
4. Decreased venous return and cardiac output
5. Fluid retention
6. Right-sided heart failure

PEEP or CPAP complications

1. Barotrauma
2. Decreased venous return and cardiac output
3. Fluid retention
4. Right heart overload
5. Overdistention

There are three mechanisms with which the pulmonary system handles a bacterial challenge. The first is the physical mechanism in which the ciliary escalator is used to eliminate bacteria and particles from the upper airway. Highly effective for larger particles or bacteria that have adhered to droplets, this mechanism is frequently destroyed by infection, bypassed by resuscitative measures, or suppressed by disease or drugs.

The humoral mechanism does not have the capability of directly handling bacterial contamination. It primarily acts to enhance the capability of the cellular mechanism.

Only the cellular mechanism has been demonstrated to be capable of effectively coping with bacterial contamination. The paramount cells in this mechanism are the alveolar macrophages. They come from promonocytes in the bone marrow, which are transported as monocytes and migrate to the alveoli where they are transformed into alveolar macrophages. These are unique from other macrophages because they are only capable of aerobic metabolism and are even immunologically and enzymatically different from other macrophages. They are activated by not yet fully described mechanisms and are capable of ingesting and killing large quantities of bacteria. Their passage from the bone marrow averages 33 hours, and their average half-life is 2 to 3 weeks. Enhanced by cell-mediated immunologic mechanisms, they can be depressed by trauma, malnutrition, and drugs, including anesthetic gases. They can be almost eliminated by the administration of corticosteroids.

The function of alveolar macrophages has been shown to be depressed by a decrease in surfactant. Surfactant has been shown to decrease after a scald burn in animals, probably because of increased leakage of serum and plasma into the alveolar space. This leakage inactivates the surface active protein or surfactant phospholipid, increases the surface tension, and contributes to atelectasis, and further inhibition of the macrophages.[5,16,17]

Inhalation of an irritant such as smoke has been investigated in laboratory animals, where it results in initial activation of the alveolar macrophages. These have increased phagocytotic and killing capacity, as evidenced by in vitro tests done on the macrophages washed from the animals' tracheobronchial trees. There is also a slight increase initially in the ability of the lung to clear aerolized bacteria, but this initial enhancement is temporary, and whether pulmonary sepsis ensues depends on the animal's overall status.

Overall, in vivo research reveals that if the animal has no concomitant cutaneous burn and survives the immediate postexposure phase, it will survive. If the animal also has a small scald (i.e., 20% of total BSA), the macrophage system will fail, and the animal will succumb within a few days of pneumonitis. Similarly, it has been found in clinical studies that, if a patient has only a smoke inhalation injury without either a cutaneous burn or other severe, associated cardiopulmonary disease and if he survives the in-fire stage and does not enter the health system moribund, he usually will survive.

PREVENTION AND TREATMENT OF SEPSIS

The problem of pulmonary sepsis, like that associated with the burn wound, is one of decreased host resistance rather than the acquisition of a particularly virulent organism. The approach to health care must therefore be broad and start as soon as possible after the patient has entered the health care system. The principles to follow in preventing and treating pulmonary sepsis are as follows:

1. Reduce the total number of bacteria by reducing the amount of an inoculum
2. Try to prevent inoculation or contamination with a virulent or antibiotic-resistant bacterial strain
3. Enhance the patient's natural host defense mechanisms
4. Observe careful and thorough pulmonary respiratory therapy procedures
5. Prevent and treat burn wound sepsis
6. Give nutritional support early
7. Recognize and treat early with specific antibiotics for lung sepsis
8. Do not give steroids or other drugs that have been shown to compromise pulmonary host defense
9. Debride eschar and close burn wound early

REFERENCES

1. Bredenberg, CE, and Webb, WR: Experimental pulmonary edema, Ann Surg 189:433, 1979.
2. Comroe, JH, et al: The lung: clinical physiology and pulmonary function tests, Chicago, 1962, Year Book Medical Publishers, Inc.
3. Dressler, DP, and Skornik, WA: Eschar: a major factor in postburn pneumonia, Am J Surg 127:413, 1974.
4. Dressler, DP, and Skornik, WA: Pulmonary bacterial susceptibility in the burned rat, Ann Surg 180:221, 1974.
5. Dressler, DP, and Skornik, WA: Alveolar macrophage function in burned rats, J Trauma 14:1036, 1974.
6. Hodgkin, JE: Ventilatory assistance, Am J Surg 138:374, 1979.
7. Hunt, JL, Purdue, GF, and Gunning, T: Is tracheostomy warranted in the burn patient? Indications and contraindications, Burn Care Rehabil 7:498, 1986.
8. Lucas, CE, et al: Effect of end-expiratory pressure on total oxygen dynamics, Surg 94:643, 1983.
9. Peters, RM: Lifesaving measures in acute respiratory distress syndrome, Am J Surg 138: 368, 1979.
10. Powers, SR, Jr, et al: Physiologic consequences of positive end-expiratory pressure (PEEP) ventilation, Ann Surg 178:265, 1973.
11. Shah, DM, et al: Cardiac output and pulmonary wedge pressure: use for evaluation of fluid replacement in trauma patients, Arch Surg 112:1161, 1977.
12. Shah, DM, et al: Continuous positive airway pressure versus positive end-expiratory pressure in respiratory distress syndrome, J Thorac Cardiovasc Surg 74:557, 1977.
13. Skornik, WA, and Dressler, DP: Lung bacterial clearance in the burned rat, Ann Surg 172:837, 1970.
14. Skornik, WA, and Dressler, DP: Effect of short-term steroid therapy on lung bacterial clearance and survival in rats, Ann Surg 170: 415, 1974.
15. Skornik, WA, and Dressler, DP: Identification of a humoral alveolar macrophage enhancement factor, Physiologist 17:3, 1974.
16. Skornik, WA, and Dressler, DP: Inhibition of alveolar macrophage function by factors washed from the lungs of burned rats, J Reticuloendothel Soc 15:5a, 1974.
17. Skornik, WA, Nathan, P, and Dressler, DP: Alveolar macrophage function in immunized, burned rats, Arch Surg 108:715, 1974.
18. Vaughan, GM, et al: Cortisol and corticotropin in burned patients, J Trauma 22: 263, 1982.
19. Wanner, A, and Cutchavaree, A: Early recognition of upper airway obstruction following smoke inhalation, Am Rev Respir Dis 108: 1421, 1973.

8 Care of the Burn Wound

OVERVIEW

In 400 B.C., Hippocrates proposed using vinegar-soaked dressings to relieve the pain associated with burn injuries and oak bark solutions to tan the wound. By 1600 Fabricius, a Swiss physician, reported on the three degrees of burn injury. Around 1800 Edward Kentisk published *An Essay on Burns,* which approached the healing

Depth of burn

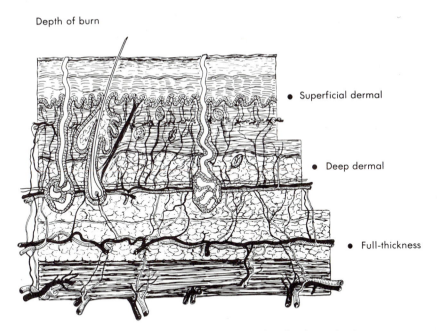

- Superficial dermal

- Deep dermal

- Full-thickness

Fig. 8-1. Schematic of normal skin showing burn depth.

of burns on a scientific basis. The first burn hospital was established by Syme in 1833 in Edinburgh and introduced the use of dry cotton wool burn dressings applied to the wound surface with firm pressure.

Varied local treatments have been used on burns: tannic acid in 1858, dressings soaked with saline in 1835, and the open treatment of burns introduced by Sneve in 1905. Davidson proposed tannic acid sprays in 1925, but this technique was abandoned due to the toxicity of the tannin. In 1937 Aldridge applied gentian violet to burns because he thought it had a bacteriostatic effect.[1a]

Despite the discovery of new antibiotics, the major reason for the remarkable progress in the treatment of burns during the past 20 years has been the description of the pathophysiology of invasive burn wound sepsis. This understanding provided the basis for the care of the burn wound described in this chapter.

STRUCTURE AND FUNCTION OF NORMAL SKIN

Fig. 8-1 shows the structure of normal skin with three degrees of burn depth. In order to appreciate the burn injury and its treatment, it is useful to start with an understanding of normal skin structure. The surface layer of the stratum corneum is generally about 15 μm thick and is composed of nonliving, dry, keratinized cells. Under the stratum corneum is the living epidermis, which is about 75 μm thick and composed of keratinocytes and some melanocytes. Cell division is limited to the basal cell layer adjacent to the dermis. Under the epidermis is the dermis, the thickness of which varies with age and body site. It is composed of interstitial collagen fibers and fibroblasts. The blood vessels and nerves in the skin run throughout the dermis but do not enter the epidermis. Hair follicles originate in the dermis. These follicles are lined with epidermal cells, which are important factors in re-epithelialization of second-degree burns. Sweat glands are also found in the dermal layer. These ducts lined with epidermal cells empty onto the skin surface. Under the dermis is the adipose tissue, which consists primarily of fat and varies in depth from barely perceptible to several inches thick.

Each layer of the skin offers special protective functions. The 25 g of stratum corneum are uniformly spread over 2 m² of the body surface. The stratum corneum controls the loss of water, electrolytes, and plasma proteins. Some water moves the epidermis by passive transport through the stratum corneum and evaporates from the body surface. The diffusion constant for water through the stratum corneum is 5×10^{-10} cm²/second, whereas through the dermis the constant is 5×10^{-6} cm²/second. The rate of water loss through skin is about 0.3 mg/cm²/hour. The average person loses about 0.25 L of water through the skin each day. Without the stratum corneum, the water loss increases to 10 mg/cm²/hour, so that in adult patients with a 50% total BSA burn of full thickness, the water loss through the surface may be 2 L/day. The fluid passing through a burn also contains electrolytes and proteins that are not lost through normal skin.[31]

The stratum corneum also serves as a barrier against bacterial invasion. Bacteria can enter hair follicles and skin glands. Bacteria normally reside on the moist skin surface of the axillae and intertriginous areas.

Destruction of the skin allows bacteria that reach the site of injury to colonize and enter the body. Local defenses include constriction of venule sphincters and clot formation. Should the bacteria not be contained, the body's immunologic system is activated to control the infection.

The stratum corneum limits the passage of foreign substances through the skin. Relatively mild injuries substantially increase the residual tissue skin permeability. Skin without a stratum corneum is quite permeable to topical drugs, including some antimicrobial agents.

PATHOPHYSIOLOGY OF THE BURN WOUND
Local effects

Skin biopsies taken in pigs 4 and 24 hours after thermal injuries (radiant heat 42 J/cm²) show progressive damage to hair follicles and dermal glands (Hinshaw, 1963).[18a] Between 24 and 48 hours there was progressive destruction of sweat glands, although the depth of burns did not increase. Similar studies in which radiant heat was applied to skin on rabbits' ears showed progressive destruction of peripheral nerve fibers during the 48 hours following injury.[19] These observations encourage prompt cooling of the burned area to limit the effects of heat on the tissue.[5,6,20,24,25,28,29]

Systemic effects

Important shifts in the fluid balance and protein occur following a large surface area burn. Microvascular permeability increases in burn tissue, and a generalized cell-membrane defect develops that results in intracellular swelling. The interstitium in burned and adjacent nonburned tissues appears to have a major role in edema formation.

Potent vasoactive mediators, including the vasoconstrictor and vasodilator prostaglandins, kinins, serotonin, histamine, oxygen radicals, and various lipid peroxides, are released from burn tissues.[21,23]

Determination of burn wound depth

The cause of the burn, presence of infection, palpation of the wound, and determination of nerve function provide useful clues in the determination of the extent and depth of the burn. Superficial or first-degree burns are characterized by a pink, moist surface after removal of a blister. The patient usually complains of a burning sensation in the wound. The area is soft and blanches readily. The burn is very sensitive to pinpricks. These wounds are covered with new epithelium in about a week. Severe sunburn, scalds from liquids less than 140° F (60° C), and some flash burns usually produce only superficial injuries.

As the depth of the burn increases, the pink surfaces change to a relatively dry, reticulated red and white surface. No burning sensation occurs, and the wound can be touched without producing any pain. Pressure sensation can be perceived, but pinpricks are no longer acutely painful. Such second-degree wounds are caused by hot, but not boiling, water; liquids that remain in contact with the surface for prolonged periods; or flash burns from explosion, hot grease, and flame burns. Some of these burns heal in 4 weeks, and others may never heal.

Patients with full-thickness or third-degree burns in which all layers of the skin have been destroyed complain of pain in peripheral areas of the injury. The burn itself is insensitive and the wound lacks elasticity. Flaming clothing, boiling water or grease, contact with hot metal, or immersion scalds generally have areas of third-degree burns.

Immersion burns of full thickness are difficult to evaluate. They may be pink or bright instead of white. These wounds, which are not painful, are dry and do not blanch with pressure.

Fourth-degree burns are thermal injuries to tissues beneath the skin. The epithelium is charred and insensitive. Molten metal, high-voltage electrical injury, prolonged contact with hot metal, and flame burns in an unconscious person suggest the possibility of fourth-degree burns.

PATHOGENESIS OF BURN WOUND SEPSIS
Scope

Burn wound sepsis, which may be locally or generally invasive, describes the level of invasive bacterial involvement of the burn wound and the adjacent tissues.

The rate and degree of invasive burn wound sepsis are factors in: the virulence of the bacteria; the number of bacteria in the inoculum or the surface of the burn wound; and the various components of the body's normal host defense mechanisms, including the degree and the percent of BSA burned, as well as all the usual mechanisms such as immunologic and cell-mediated response.[13,22,23,32,34]

Because of this relationship between virulence and the severe depletion of host defense mechanisms found in patients with a major thermal injury, death is most often the result of low, virulent, opportunistic organisms, i.e., of either bacteria or fungi. This finding is similar to the problems associated with opportunistic organisms in those patients receiving immunosuppression for cancer chemotherapy or organ transplants or in those patients in whom the immune system is depressed as a result of the virus that causes acquired immune deficiency syndrome (AIDS).

Natural history of sepsis

Examination of the burn wound shows that many of the wounds are relatively free of bacteria during the first 24 hours following injury. Within 3 days postburn, surface colonization increases, and bacterial proliferation occurs into the depths of the hair follicles. At this early stage gram-positive cocci, primarily the staphylococci, predominate, but some gram-negative organisms can be identified. The colonizing cells spread from the base of the hair follicles and, by the fourth or fifth day postburn, extensive involvement of the wound develops. At this time *Pseudomonas aeruginosa* and other gram-negative organisms may begin to predominate in the wound. Bacteria in large numbers permeate the burn wound and invasion occurs.

Fig. 8-2 shows the relationship of the numbers of *P. aeruginosa* per gram of subeschar tissue to the mortality rate in rats with 20% BSA having third-degree burn. With this amount of burn, at 1 billion (10^9) bacteria per gram, the mortality rate was only 63%. This would increase if either the burn area were larger or the bacteria more virulent. Conversely, a bacteria or fungus of lesser virulence might not cause death at all, unless there were other reasons that adversely affect the host defense mechanisms.[30]

Some investigators believe that bacteria may survive deep in the crypts of sweat glands and hair follicles. Initially, some colonization of the wound occurs, primarily by staphylococci, on the second or third day following injury. Rapid multiplication occurs with spreading invasive infection, including *Pseudomonas, Proteus,* and other gram-negative organisms, and staphylococci. Later, staphylococci are displaced by gram-negative flora.[9,27]

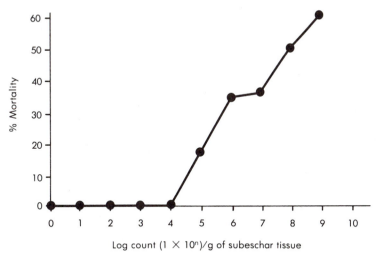

Mortality rate vs. subeschar bacterial colony count in seeded and nonseeded nontreated animals

Log count (1×10^n)/g of subeschar tissue

Fig. 8-2. Mortality rate vs. subeschar bacterial counts.

Another source of infection is the external contamination of wounds. Surface contamination occurs, particularly in the areas of the buttocks and inner thighs. In these areas fecal flora abound. Bacteria may gain access to the wound from unsterile dressings and instruments or from the respiratory or intestinal tract of the patient or attendants. A concerted effort should also be made to avoid cross contamination between patients.

Burn wound sepsis was defined by Teplitz and associates[34] as bacteria growing in the burn wound containing 100,000 bacteria per gram of eschar and involving adjacent normal tissues. Emphasis is on the large numbers of bacteria; and sepsis is differentiated from colonization, which does not involve normal tissue and is a more benign process. Frequently the infection appears to be largely concentrated in and around the wound. Therefore considerable effort should be expended toward control of the bacteria in the wound.

Invasive sepsis is initially spotty and only later becomes confluent. Moisture greatly favors the process, as is seen in the dependent areas of a patient who is not turned and in the wet, constantly approximated upper medial thighs. In contrast, the anterior trunk, a usually dry area, may remain free of detectable bacteria. Fig. 8-3 shows an obese patient with a hot water burn extending from the anterior trunk down to the anterior and medial thighs. Such patients rapidly become septic unless intensive local care is instituted even during the shock phase.

Burn wound sepsis as found in the early postburn period occurs most frequently in patients who sustain extensive, full-thickness burns. When the wounds have

anxiety and stress of being involved in a fire. In like manner, the occurrence of cerebral ischemia from whatever cause may further contribute to the injury by prolonging exposure to toxic gases or heat.

Early physical signs include: (1) development of rales and inspiratory stridor caused by upper airway obstruction or bronchospasm, and (2) expiratory stridor indicative of upper airway obstruction and severe bronchospasm caused by edema and inhalation of an irritant or the inhalation of substances to which the patient is allergic. Both findings, particularly expiratory stridor, demand immediate treatment. Early onset of hoarseness and vocal cord lesions may be the result of nonspecific irritants or acid particulate matter. Stupor or unconsciousness, facial burns, singed nasal vibrissae, bronchorrea, and sooty sputum are also pathognomonic.[30,44,52,67,83]

LABORATORY STUDIES
pH and blood gases

No one test has more diagnostic value than the determination of arterial blood pH and gases. Ventilation and perfusion abnormalities (i.e., blood-gas values and xenon 133 lung scan studies) can precede clinically apparent hypoxemia. Generally, a Pa_{O_2} of less than 75 torr is diagnostic. A marked metabolic acidosis also exists in at least one half of all cases studied.[49,58,78,79]

As a result of recent advances in equipment development, most hospitals can readily and accurately determine arterial blood pH and gases. Some confusion may exist whether the sample is arterial, or there may be difficulty in performing the arterial puncture in a severely burned patient, particularly in a patient in shock, but the puncture can usually be accomplished from the femoral artery, even at the risk of transcending burn tissue and before considerable edema has developed.

Once the diagnosis has been made or confirmed and it appears that repeat or frequent determinations will either be required or difficult, a catheter can be placed in a convenient artery, preferably the radial; but even the femoral artery should not be ruled out in a risk/benefit evaluation.

Although it may appear that the simple identification of abnormalities in pH or blood gas values may establish the diagnosis, a number of pitfalls exist. The determination may be made too early following exposure, abnormalities may be a result of obstruction of the airway, or metabolic disturbances related to shock may occur. The patient may also have other nonassociated cardiopulmonary diseases related to or independent of the present injury, or there may be late-term toxicologic effects caused by the inhalation of a product of combustion. Despite these pitfalls, these tests are critical because the treatment is usually nonspecific as it relates to the etiology and is directly related to the maintenance of normal pH and blood gas levels.

Hypoxemia, significant if present, may initially be absent in 80% of patients who subsequently develop evidence of inhalation damage. Pulmonary dysfunction occurs with an increase in alveolar-arterial P_{O_2} gradient and a decrease in compliance.

Pulmonary function

A number of pulmonary function tests exist that are generally nonspecific and related more to the irritant properties of a given pyrolysate and its subsequent edema formation. Although these tests may be of benefit in long-term assessment and care, they offer little additional information over a basic history and physical examination with continued monitoring of the patient, including determination of blood gases. It should be noted that, in evaluating most inhalation exposure victims, baseline data are usually not available. In a thoracic cage burn with the subsequent development of edema and decreased compliance, pulmonary resistance tests can be as high as four times normal, and compliance can be reduced by more than 50%. If smoke inhalation is suspected, the most valuable pulmonary function tests can be those that are repeated, following either initial observation or treatment.[33,57,63,74,85]

Special studies

Special studies refer to tests such as sputum cytology[2,28] and specific tests for neurotoxic, hepatoxic, and nephrotoxic effects. Extravascular lung water studies show an increase in vascular shunting and extravascular water, but these results are of little value in diagnosis, prognosis, or treatment. On the basis of present information, these tests are recommended only as part of a research protocol. However, it is strongly recommended that as many toxicologic screening tests as possible be obtained, including those for blood alcohol and legal and illegal drugs, particularly in the patient who is critically ill or in whom the diagnosis or management is not clear. Even under optimum circumstances several days can elapse before test results are available. At this time, treatment enigmas can often be explained by the results seen in the patient's condition. Therefore the present role of specific chemical tissue tests is limited to forensic, research, or occupational medicine.[9,19,84]

RADIOLOGIC EVALUATION
Chest x-ray film

Although a routine chest x-ray film finding that shows a generalized ground glass effect consistent with edema of the large and small bronchi is probably caused by the inhalation of irritants, this diagnosis is ordinarily made from 12 to 14 hours following exposure, well after it should be made if prompt treatment is to be instituted. A chest x-ray film should be made in the emergency room by means of a portable machine to determine the presence of other injuries or the existence of associated cardiopulmonary disease.[14]

Later, often enroute to the in-hospital bed, a more extensive in-department chest x-ray film is recommended, at which time the position of the airways, CVP, and other long lines can be determined. This also serves as a baseline for future studies.

Customarily the policy is to radiograph the chests of all individuals who may have been exposed to smoke. This often involves large numbers of fire fighters. Standard chest x-ray films are wasteful and generally unrewarding during the early phases following exposure, unless some physical findings are present.

Routine admission chest x-ray films are mandatory; these are needed to check for long line positions, possible pneumothorax following long line insertion, development of atelectasis, cardiac failure, sepsis, and the presence or absence of associated cardiopulmonary disease. These procedures are safe and do not necessarily require patient cooperation.

Xenon 133 lung scan

Another radiologic procedure generally accepted to be 95% accurate for the determination of smoke inhalation injury is the xenon 133 lung scanning study. This test traces the diffusion of the xenon 133 through the pulmonary or alveolar capillaries and through the alveolar membrane into the alveolar space. Thus any thickening from edema fluid in the space between the endothelium and the alveolar membrane such as occurs from the inhalation of a pulmonary irritant can be noted early following exposure, depending on the dosage and type of pyrolysate.[56]

Later, inactivation of the surfactant, especially the loss of capillary permeability, can result in abnormal findings. Loss of capillary permeability can also occur with a cutaneous burn alone as a result of the development of acute respiratory distress syndrome (ARDS) or from iatrogenic causes, which can confuse the findings. These latter etiologic factors can emerge within hours, but they usually emerge, at the earliest, 12 hours following injury, thus allowing for a valid and early xenon 133 study. Since resuscitation and subsequent treatment are based more on physical findings and blood gases than on xenon 133 scanning studies, these isotope studies should not be performed if they would delay or impede treatment. However, they are highly valuable prognostic indicators.

Procedure. The xenon 133 in saline is not readily available but can be obtained on standing order from a radiopharmaceutical firm. Standard equipment is used throughout the procedure. The standard perfusion scan performed with macroaggregated albumin does not demonstrate smoke inhalation injury. The patient is positioned with his anterior thorax against a gamma camera, and 10 to 20 mCi of xenon 133 in saline solution is injected intravenously. Virtually all xenon 133 in the bolus will enter the alveolar air spaces during its first transit. Sequential scintiphotographs obtained every 30 seconds will monitor regional washout of xenon 133 from alveoli.

Findings. Fig. 9-1 shows the normal distribution of xenon 133 in the lung at various times following injection through the right subclavian vein. It can be noted that at 0 to 6 seconds there is a high concentration in the right subclavian vein, and there is a high homogeneous distribution throughout the lung at the 6- to 12-second

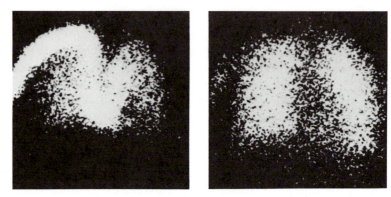

0-6 Seconds   6-12 Seconds

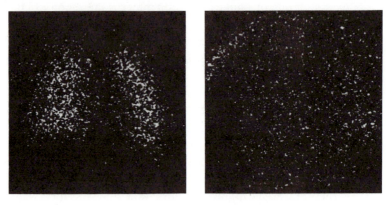

30-60 Seconds   90-120 Seconds

Fig. 9-1. Normal xenon-133 lung diffusion scan. (Courtesy Col. Robert J. Lull, MC USA, Letterman Army Medical Center, Presidio of San Francisco, Calif.)

interval. By the 30- to 60-second time period, there is a rapid and even clearing, which is almost complete by 90 to 120 seconds.

In contrast, in the patient with a smoke inhalation injury (Fig. 9-2), in which the injection has been given through the inferior vena caval system, a delay in clearing of the xenon 133 and a distinct regional trapping of the gas occur. The change in injection site is the reason for the nonvisualization of the subclavian vein.

These findings can be confused with atelectasis or chronic obstructive pulmonary disease (COPD). In cases involving atelectasis a delay of up to several days usually occurs; therefore this does not detract from the value of the test during the critical early postburn period; like all tests, the need exists to evaluate it in context with other findings. Since 80% of the positive patients will return to normal by the fourth

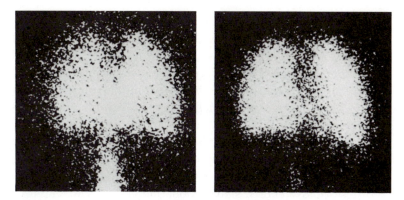

0-6 Seconds   6-12 Seconds

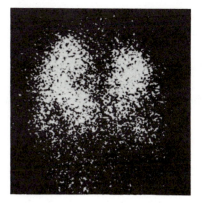 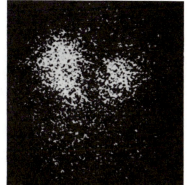

30-60 Seconds   150-180 Seconds

Fig. 9-2. Xenon-133 lung diffusion scan in patient with smoke inhalation injury. (Courtesy Col. Robert J. Lull, MC USA, Letterman Army Medical Center, Presidio of San Francisco, Calif.)

day, a delay in obtaining this test may also result in a false-negative result. In the case of COPD, the diagnostic nonspecificity of xenon 133 is not unique to this situation but to some degree pertains to all lung studies.

Fiberoptic bronchoscopy

Indications. This simple procedure has been shown to be approximately 90% accurate in making the diagnosis of smoke inhalation injury. Unfortunately, a positive finding does not necessarily correlate with the severity of the injury. What is actually being demonstrated is: (1) the effect of heat on the upper airway with possible obstruction as a result of edema, and (2) the effect of irritants on the bronchi, also with swelling caused by edema and the presence of soot particles, thereby further raising the suspicion of inhalation injury. Although these determinations could possibly just as easily and accurately be made with a thorough physical examination of the oropharynx, the ease, minimal risk, and low cost of this procedure does make it worthwhile. What the fiberoptic bronchoscope does not show is possible damage to the small or terminal bronchi and the alveoli.

Technique. Any of the commonly available equipment in an emergency room is usually adequate to perform fiberoptic bronchoscopy. Topical anesthetic should be used if necessary. The importance of doing a complete examination of the oropharynx should be emphasized. This procedure should be performed after patient resuscitative efforts, stabilization, and case review. The decision to treat depends more on suspicion and requires immediate attention to cardiopulmonary resuscitation, including airway provision, ventilatory support and oxygen, followed by blood gases and treatment of specific imbalances. The fiberoptoscope is more helpful in prognosis and planning treatment than in diagnosis.

Findings. Depending on the degree and duration of exposure and the time since extrication, varying amounts of edema, erythema, soot particles, mucosal necrosis, or even charring will occur. Although the degree of severity of these findings will correlate somewhat with the prognosis, the main purpose and benefit from this procedure is the detection of any degree of injury so that arterial blood samples and full respiratory support can be started promptly.

SELECTED ETIOLOGIC FACTORS

A number of specific etiologic factors exist that have a direct bearing on the acute effects of smoke inhalation in humans. These factors, together with the sources and physiologic effects of selected thermodecomposition gases, are presented in Table 9-1.[59,84]

Oxygen depletion and effects of hypoxia

As typically shown in the analysis of a small-scale test (Fig. 9-3), as well as in large-scale tests, oxygen depletion occurs in any fire, even without the occurrence of a flashover. Concomitantly, carbon monoxide and carbon dioxide increase.[23,24]

Incidence. Hypoxia is frequent and can be related to many causes, either directly a result of the injury or secondary to shock, with or without inhalation exposure. Another important consideration is the patient's medical condition such as myocardial infarction or a disease entity existing before exposure and aggravated by the fire. Also not to be missed are effects of other injuries that may have occurred at the time, but can be overlooked because of the dramatic appearance or pain of the fire victim.

The signs and symptoms of hypoxia (Table 9-2) can range from a subtle loss of fine and color vision to complete collapse and rapid death.[51,88]

Table 9-1. Sources and physiologic effects of selected thermodecomposition gases other than CO and CO_2

Gas	Sources	Highlights of physiologic effect	Estimated 10-minute lethal concentration (ppm)
Hydrogen cyanide (HCN)	Wool, silk, polyacrylonitrile, nylon, polyurethane, paper	Rapidly fatal histoxic asphyxia No definite data	350
Nitrogen dioxide (NO_2) and other oxides of nitrogen	Cellulose nitrate	Irritant, immediate death and delayed injury	> 200
Ammonia (NH_3)	Wool, silk, nylon, melamine	Pungent odor, high irritant	> 1000
Hydrogen chloride (HCl)	PVC, chlorinate acrylics, retardant materials	Respiratory irritant, potential toxicity of HCl on particles greater than gaseous HCl	> 500
Other halogen acid gases	Fluorinated resins or films, bromine, fire retardants	Respiratory irritants	HF: 400 COF2: 100 HBr: > 500
Sulfur dioxide (SO_2)	Sulfur compounds	Intolerable well below lethal levels	> 500
Isocyanates	Urethane isocyanates, occurrence in real fires undetermined	Potent respiratory irritant	> 100
Acrolein	Polyolefins, cellulose, major irritant from wood	Potent respiratory irritant	30-100

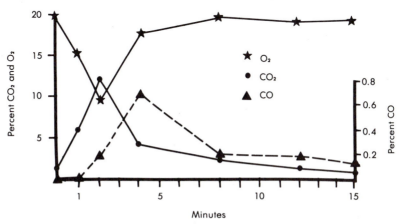

Fig. 9-3. Chamber analysis for oxygen, carbon monoxide, and carbon dioxide following ignition of white pine wood.

Table 9-2. Signs and symptoms of reduced levels of oxygen due to fires

Oxygen (%)	Sign or symptom
15-17	Loss of fine and color vision
12-15	Loss of muscular and skilled movement and coordination
10-14	Faulty judgment
6-8	Rapid collapse
0-6	Death in 1 to 6 minutes

Diagnosis

Clinical. Although the signs and symptoms associated with respiratory distress such as rapid and often shallow respiration, increased pulse rate and blood pressure, and especially anxiety and apprehension occur frequently, in burn patients the possibility of decreased compliance as a result of a burn of the chest wall exists.

Laboratory. The laboratory diagnosis of hypoxia confirms clinical impression, since at this stage the treatment should have already commenced on the basis of history and clinical findings. The results, however, are invaluable in subsequently managing the patient.

Treatment. The basic principles of treatment include cardiopulmonary resuscitation, ventilatory and respiratory support, and correction of metabolic acidosis (i.e., the oxygen dissociation curve which also includes correction of hemoglobin deficits). Treatment should be continued until the patient can maintain normal blood gases without assisted respiratory support.

Carbon monoxide

Incidence. Extensive investigations have shown carbon monoxide to be the major toxicant in deaths from smoke inhalation. The toxicity of carbon monoxide is a result of the formation of blood carboxyhemoglobin (COHb), which results in the reduced ability of the blood to transport oxygen (Table 9-3). Extremely dangerous ranges of carbon monoxide, usually several thousand parts per million, are commonly found in the fire environment. Even a lesser amount can be lethal, depending on the duration of exposure and associated impaired cardiopulmonary function. COHb levels of 4% to 6% have been shown to increase the threshold for ventricular fibrillation in normal dogs. Combinations of elevated COHb with drugs or alcohol can be even more deadly in shorter exposure periods.[26,29,73,80,94-96]

The signs and symptoms at various concentrations of carboxyhemoglobin are displayed in Table 9-4. It is interesting to note that smokers have a COHb level of 5%, whereas traffic police may have 15% to 20%. The presence of malfunctioning furnaces are undoubtedly the cause of many undiagnosed chronic headaches.

Table 9-3. Carbon monoxide response

CO concentration (ppm)	Response
100	Allowable for several hours
400-500	No appreciable effect after 1 hour
600-700	Just appreciable after 1 hour
1000-1200	Unpleasant after 1 hour
1500-2000	Dangerous when inhaled for 1 hour
4000	Fatal at less than 1 hour
10,000	Fatal at 1 minute

Table 9-4. Signs and symptoms at various concentrations of carboxyhemoglobin (COHb)

COHb (%)	Signs and symptoms
10-19	Slight headache, dilation of vessels
20-29	Headache
30-39	Headache, weakness, loss of visual acuity, nausea and vomiting, and collapse
40-49	Greater incidence of collapse, increased pulse and respiration
50-59	Coma, convulsions, Cheyne-Stokes respiration
60-69	Convulsions, decreased heart and respiratory rates, possible death
70-79	Slow respiration, moribund
80-89	Death in less than 1 hour
90 +	Death in less than 1 minute

Diagnosis

Clinical. The clinical signs may vary from mild respiratory distress, mental abnormalities, and agitation to coma. If oxygen has been given, it is important that the half-life of COHb be calculated, particularly after treatment, so that less obvious clinical signs are not missed.

Laboratory. This test is essentially a COHb determination. It can be performed most rapidly using any standard photometric method that is generally accurate to within 5% to 10% and is fully satisfactory in diagnosing, treating, and monitoring the patient. The ease, availability, and cost make it even more acceptable. Hyperamylasemia with levels sometimes exceeding 1000 Somogyi units have been reported with only carbon monoxide poisoning.[81] The finding of hyperamylasemia may or may not be helpful in the diagnosis of carbon monoxide, but the amylase level is not related to survival and requires no treatment.

Treatment. Treatment is full ventilatory and respiratory support with high levels of oxygen. With the optimum ventilation and the use of 100% oxygen, the half-life of COHb is 30 to 40 minutes. In room air, the half-life is 4 to 5 hours. Hyperbaric oxygen (HBO) may make a difference in survival if it is available immediately. In actual practice, the prompt implementation of 100% oxygen at the scene accompanied by efficient ventilatory support has been shown to be equally effective. It is generally believed that active treatment should be continued until the COHb level is below 5% to fully treat any possible long-term mental sequelae.

Prognosis. If the patient is not moribund and has no other extenuating injuries or diseases, with treatment he or she will usually survive an acute exposure to carbon monoxide. Long-term neurologic deficits do occur, however, and should be cited.

Pulmonary irritants

Source and type. Pulmonary irritants are some of the most common products of combustion outside of carbon monoxide and carbon dioxide. They can be severely irritating. Such irritants include aldehydes, the acrolein produced from the combustion of wood or wood products, and halogenated synthetic polymers such as polyvinyl chloride (PVC)[10,17,32,87] and polytetrafluoroethylene (PTFE or TEFLON).[13,15,71,72,89] PVC combines with water to form hydrochloric acid (HCl), and PTFE degrades to carbon dioxide (CO_2) and hydrogen fluoride (HF). When heated, PVC does not degrade or unzip to the monomer vinyl chloride, which on prolonged exposure is carcinogenic. It does, however, produce a highly irritating HCl. This pyrolysate, like those from PTFE, primarily is given off at temperatures well below the ignition temperature, often before visible smoke is observed. Although HCl can be produced in small-scale laboratory tests, in full-scale tests less than 2% of the stoichiometric predictable HCl can be identified, probably because of the highly adherent and hydroscopic properties of HCl. It is problematic whether this material is a severe hazard in actual fires unless the highly unusual circumstance of an electrical power room fire occurs with massive exposure to an unsuspecting victim. In this case, massive, rapid upper and lower respiratory tract edema could be fatal. Some question exists as to whether the HCl adhering to water droplets or particulate matter is small enough (i.e., >5 μm) to enter and damage the lower tract.

PVC was developed for the U.S. Navy in World War II because it does not ignite or support combustion. Many of the toxicity properties that have been attributed to it may be caused by the plasticizers, stabilizers, coloring agents, or other chemicals in the polymer, which can account for as much as 55% of a commercial PVC product. COF2, COF$_3$, and CF4 are also major pyrolysates of PTFE, but it is doubtful whether these are important outside of the laboratory.

Effect

Clinical. Diagnosis for smoke inhalation is readily made with complaints of eye tearing, burning of the nose and throat, and other irritating effects, but the significance of the inhalation injury depends on the development of and the degree of the response and the location. If localized to the upper airway, the clinical signs and symptoms should be directed to obstructions, particularly of the larynx. Stridor can develop. The exposure of the lower bronchi to the irritant is not frequent, but it is not unusual; the clinical signs are the development of rales and rhonchi, often occurring 10 to 12 hours after exposure and usually subsiding in 24 hours. In practice, if a patient has not developed any clinical signs within 2 to 3 hours following exposure, it is doubtful if signs will appear at a later time. In rare instances a patient is exposed to a massive dose of an irritant, and, before rescue can be attempted, death may occur from a massive and rapid upper airway obstruction caused by asphyxiation. In these cases the diagnosis is obvious, although nonspecific. If the victim is rescued alive, the treatment is immediate airway relief and ventilation. As a result of the etiology and circumstances of the death, postmortem findings cannot identify a specific causative agent.

   Laboratory. The laboratory findings following exposure to a pulmonary irritant are nonspecific. They are related more to the effects of the pulmonary edema. It is doubtful whether any of the irritants directly affect any component of the acid/base system or whether the agents can be detected by tissue studies.

OTHER PRODUCTS OF COMBUSTION
Carbon dioxide

   Carbon dioxide has long been thought to be innocuous and not a factor in inhalation injury. Although it is well accepted that in small amounts it is a respiratory stimulant, which therefore could contribute to the more rapid inhalation of other toxic products, it is also a depressant at higher levels, thus further preventing victims from escaping. Although these factors might in themselves demonstrate the importance of this common product of combustion, carbon dioxide has also been shown to contribute to abnormal acid/base findings when inhaled at the levels and duration commonly found in fires. These levels can be as high as 15%, but, when lower, they are commonly associated with more deadly increases in carbon monoxide levels.

Water

   Water, in greatly varying amounts, is also a frequent product of combustion. However, it has been well demonstrated that a higher content of water in inhaled smoke will result in a higher temperature in the respiratory tract and increased absorption of products. Unlike the inhalation of steam with its superheated qualities, water is not a substantial factor in smoke inhalation, except that water droplets may serve as a vehicle for the transport of absorbed acids such as HCl.

Heat

Since the studies of Moritz and Henriques[53] and Moritz, Henriques, and McLean,[54] heat has generally not been thought to be a major factor in inhalation injury. However, it is a factor in injury to the oropharynx, and the massive inhalation of hot gases can result in rapid massive edema with obstruction and death. In those victims who survive the fire and are seen in an emergency facility, alive and not moribund, this obstruction usually develops over several hours. With this knowledge, suitable airways can be placed to preclude any obstruction, pending the subsiding of the edema after the shock phase and during the diuretic phase. In rats heat probably contributes to the toxicity of inhaled products because of increased respiration and/ or metabolism. Though a logical assumption, this has been difficult to prove in humans.

Particulate matter

Particulate matter, the visible component of smoke, is by definition visible and therefore larger than 5 μm in size. At this size, however, the particles are too large to reach the alveoli. Therefore their role in producing an inhalation injury is debatable, though they certainly contribute to the opacity of the environment and add to the stress and the other factors obstructing escape. They also serve as a visible warning, trigger alarm systems, and thus aid in early escape. Also, the presence of particulate matter (e.g., soot) in the upper airway can serve as an indicator of some degree of inhalation injury and therefore can be indirectly beneficial. Some investigators hypothesize that certain hydroscopic pyrolysates such as HCl can adhere to these particles and thus be transported to some level in the tracheorespiratory tree where they can directly cause damage, increase edema, and even result in late sequelae. It is estimated from laboratory models that less than 2% of the amount of predicted HCl produced is absorbed on the soot. How much of this reaches the lower airway is arguable. During the early stages of a fire when escape is most possible, the gas that is not seen is probably more dangerous than the smoke with particles that can be seen (Table 9-5).

Table 9-5. Smoke analysis of several common materials

Toxic compound	Wood	Kerosene	Cotton	MAC* (ppm)
Acrolein	50	1	60	0.1
Formaldehyde	80	10	70	5
Acetaldehyde	200	60	120	200
Butyraldehyde	100	1	7	—

*MAC, Maximum allowable industrial concentration.

Hydrogen cyanide

Hydrogen cyanide is more toxic than carbon monoxide. It poisons the tissue respiration by reacting with the Fe III of the cytochrome oxidase, thereby preventing the use of oxygen by tissues. Theoretically it can be produced during the pyrolysis of all natural or synthetic polymers containing nitrogen.

In actual practice only small amounts of hydrogen cyanide are produced, and its clinical significance is difficult to establish.[19,36-38,43] Toxic levels of cyanide have been found in victims of airplane crashes. However, the validity of hydrogen cyanide tests is open to question for the following reasons: (1) the body produces this chemical both in the living and postmortem tissue, (2) tests are difficult to perform, and (3) they have been made up to several weeks after the incident.

Hydrogen cyanide, a histotoxic agent, should be in greater concentrations than 1 μg/ml before significant toxicologic effects can be attributed to its presence. Blood levels above 3 μg are lethal. It is unknown at what stage of the fire development, or more specifically, at what point in the fire dynamics related to the production of other products and circumstances that preclude escape that the hydrogen cyanide has been produced.

Nitrates and nitrites

These compounds have well-known adverse effects on the cardiovascular system. They are produced during the off-gas phase and during the combustion of polymethylacrylate (Plexiglas).[37] A dense black smoke is produced, but during the off-gas phase the smoke is colorless. In the laboratory this can rapidly cause death in rats before the smoke becomes visible. It is difficult to sort out this effect in fire victims, considering all the later events that occur. Levels directly or even indirectly derived from some admixture of the oxides of nitrogen in the form of methemoglobin (metHb) have not been reported except in several cases in which patients have been treated topically with silver nitrate solution in a report by Schwerd and Schulz[73] in Germany in 1978. This finding, metHb, theoretically should be more common and may represent a major toxic factor that has not yet been adequately investigated.

Aliphatic and aromatic hydrocarbons

Theoretically all hydrocarbons, when inhaled, have an anesthetic or narcotic effect. In clinical practice these properties have been enhanced by halogenation to produce anesthetic agents such as halothane, which can be hepatotoxic. This could have far reaching, deadly effects when inhaled in a fire (Table 9-6). In addition to the narcotic effect, the aromatic hydrocarbons have varying irritating properties. Some, like benzene, can be absorbed through the skin. Although their presence is not uncommon in a fire, unless there are unusual circumstances or in industry or ware-

Table 9-6. Common aliphatic and aromatic hydrocarbons

Compound	MAC (ppm)*
Propane	1000
Butane	1000
Hexane	500
Heptane	500
Octane	500
1,3-Butadiene	1000
Benzene	100
Styrene	100

*MAC, Maximum allowable industrial concentration.

housing, the concentrations are minimal and insignificant in proportion to other pyrolysates.

Free radicals

Recently, considerable attention has been paid to the presence of stable free radicals in the combustion products. These free radicals have been identified in concentrations of up to 1200 ppm in fire environments in which the carbon monoxide level has not exceeded 500 ppm. It has been shown in the laboratory that unidentified but stable free radicals can cause rapid incapacitation by lipid peroxidation of the pulmonary surfactant, resulting in a rapid increase of surface tension and concomitant hypoxia. The presence of free radicals also enhances carbon monoxide asphyxia and relates directly to the inhibition of the alveolar macrophages, thereby contributing to the major cause of death, pulmonary sepsis.[82]

Materials may reproduce free radicals during the off-gas phase and therefore may be toxic without the occurrence of combustion. The full impact of free radical toxicity has yet to be fully investigated or accepted, but it does portend the need for development of specific preventive and therapeutic methods.[12,50,61,91]

Other products

Infrequent products of combustion are: sulfur dioxide; nitrogen dioxide and other oxides of nitrogen; ammonia (NH_3); isocyanates; and heavy metals such as antimony, zinc, and chromium. Antimony has frequently been used in fire retardants but has not yet been demonstrated to be a major factor in inhalation injury. Some of the earlier fire retardants used in children's pajama fabrics are possibly carcinogenic, but that is not within the scope of smoke toxicology. Also not within the scope, but most important to consider, is the inhalation of toxic chemicals by workers or fire fighter personnel who become exposed to chemicals released in an industrial accident.[4,11,25,39,46,68,75,93]

Synthetic products rarely consist of single polymers, but usually contain additives as stabilizers, plasticizers, fillers, and coloring agents. It is not unusual that a manufacturer is unable to identify all of the additives in a commercial product. Fortunately, most of these additives are small in amount and relatively nontoxic, or their adverse effect is miniscule in comparison to other materials in the product or environment.

Some additives such as the various phosphorus additives will need continued testing to identify the unusually toxic chemical. Although these hazardous findings receive considerable publicity (e.g., one of the over 300 available polyurethane foams now off the market because of thermal degradation, a bicyclophosphate ester, or nerve gas), many remain to be identified by those in toxicology or occupational medicine. In clinical practice it is advisable to be aware of the potential hazards, to evaluate them judiciously, and, in diagnosing and treating the smoke inhalation victim, to maintain an overall perspective of the complex fire scene and resultant injuries.

TREATMENT
Specific

Theoretically some inhaled pyrolysates have specific antidotes such as those for hydrogen cyanide. However, the rarity of their occurrence, the difficulty in their identification, and the inherent time delay on the basis of present knowledge precludes the use of any specific therapy for smoke inhalation, with the exception of oxygen for carbon monoxide, which therapeutic modality is also a component of nonspecific therapy.

Nonspecific

All treatment of miscellaneous inhaled pyrolysates is nonspecific, including respiratory support. Understanding the mechanisms will help in the treatment, planning, and prognosis. A clear airway with adequate ventilatory and respiratory support is mandatory. Maintenance of a clear airway and correction of common metabolic acidosis can best be accomplished with serial determinations of arterial pH and blood gases. Judicious fluid therapy is also critical; administration of fluids can be exceedingly difficult if there is some degree of cardiogenic shock.[7,67,78]

Respiratory support

The chapter on respiratory care discusses PEEP and CPAP and airways in detail. Bronchodilators, oxygen, and corrections of acid/base imbalance are also common therapeutic modalities that should be monitored closely. The need for blood transfusion is rare and only indicated with a preexisting disease or an associated injury, particularly since the use of an oropharyngeal or nasopharyngeal airway and the presence of bronchorrhea markedly alter the physical mechanism of the pulmonary bacterial host defense system and the alveolar macrophage system, which may be diminished. Accordingly, the tracheobronchial tract must be kept as clean as possible. This requires frequent suction, often with lavage, and encouragement of the patient's own respiratory efforts.[20,60,66,74,76]

Steroids

Steroids have often been given to the burn patient to reduce the capillary alveolar permeability and also to reduce bronchospasm that results primarily from the inhalation of an irritant. In the laboratory massive doses of corticosteroids such as dexamethasone and methylprednisolone have been shown to be effective in this latter area; but the mineralocorticosteroids such as cortisone and hydrocortisone have increased mortality. Unfortunately, even one massive dose of these agents can effectively reduce or eliminate the number of alveolar macrophages washed from the lungs and make a laboratory animal more susceptible to the inhalation of a bacterial suspension.

Since the major cause of morbidity and mortality in inhalation injury, as well as in cutaneous burn patients, is pulmonary sepsis and because many other bronchodilators that work as well or better than corticosteroids are available, there is no reason to give corticosteroids to a victim of smoke inhalation or to a burn patient. Complete adrenal depletion is a rarity, particularly during the immediate postburn period.[22]

Antibiotics

Prophylactic antibiotics are not recommended. Sputum cultures and Gram stains should be obtained on admission and repeated daily as indicated. Antibiotics should be selected on a specific basis with a plan for treating existing infections.

PROGNOSIS

The prognosis can vary markedly because the course of smoke inhalation injury is unpredictable. However, some general patterns exist. The first is airway obstruction, then pulmonary insufficiency, followed by a period, lasting a few days, of increased pulmonary bacterial susceptibility. How these issues, together with the complications caused by the pulmonary effects of other injuries or diseases, can be dealt with clinically will largely influence the outcome.

As expected, there is a substantial correlation between age and the prognosis. An even more important correlation is between the percent of total BSA burn and the prognosis. The nonmoribund patient without a concomitant cutaneous burn rarely dies. In determining the probability of survival, the dose exposure vs. mortality curve reveals that the outcome shifts with age and with the presence or absence of other disease entities or injuries, including the presence of a cutaneous burn.

In a patient with a smoke inhalation injury, data for making a prognosis are only available for the short-term effects of an acute single exposure. Although data are not available regarding long-term effects, it is reasonable to assume that some significant effect exists, particularly in those cases with extensive sloughing of the bronchial mucosa or the development of sepsis. These effects are probably in the form of pulmonary fibrosis, which can also relate to the long-established sequelae caused by stenosis at a tracheostomy site, erosion from long-term tube use, and pulmonary fibrosis from inhalation of irritants and/or pneumonitis.

REFERENCES

1. Alarie, Y, et al: Toxicity of thermal decomposition products: an attempt to correlate results obtained in small scale with large scale test, J Comb Toxicol 8:58, 1981.
2. Ambiavargar, M, Chalon, J, and Zargham, I: Tracheobronchial cytologic changes following lower airway thermal injury: a preliminary report, J Trauma 14:280, 1974.
3. Aub, JC, and Pittman, H: Management of Cocoanut Grove burns at the Massachusetts General Hospital. The pulmonary complications: a clinical description, Ann Surg 117: 834, 1943.
4. Autian, J: Toxicological aspects of flammability and combustion of polymeric materials, J Fire Flammabil 1:239, 1970.
5. Aviado, DM, and Schmidt, CF: Respiratory burns with special reference to pulmonary edema and congestion, Circulation 6:666, 1962.
6. Axford, AT, et al: Accidental exposure to isocyanate fumes in a group of firemen, Br J Ind Med 33:65, 1976.
7. Bartlett, RH, et al: Acute management of the upper airway in facial burns and smoke inhalation, Arch Surg 111:744, 1976.
8. Best, RL: Tragedy in Kentucky, Fire J 210:18, 1978.
9. Birky, MM: Philosophy of testing for assessment of toxicological aspects of fire exposure, J Comb Toxicol 3:5, 1976.
10. Boettner, EA, Ball, G, and Weiss, B: Analysis of the volatile combustion product of vinyl plastics, J Appl Polymer Sci 13:377, 1969.
11. Brown, JE, and Birky, MM: Phosgene in the thermal decomposition products of poly(vinyl chloride): generation, detection and measurement, J Anal Toxicol 4:166, 1980.
12. Buckley, GB: The role of oxygen-free radicals in human disease processes, Surgery 94:407, 1983.
13. Carter, VL, Jr, et al: The acute inhalation toxicology in rats from pyrolysis products of four fluoropolymers, Toxicol Appl Pharmacol 30: 369, 1974.
14. Clark, WR, et al: Positive computed tomography of dog lungs following severe smoke inhalation: diagnosis of inhalation injury, J Burn Care 3:207, 1982.
15. Coleman, WE, Scheel, LD, and Gorski, CH: The particles resulting from polytetrafluoroethylene (PTFF) pyrolysis in air, Am Ind Hyg Assoc J 29:54, 1968.
16. Cope, O, and Rhinelander, FW: The problem of burn shock complicated by pulmonary damage, Ann Surg 117:915, 1943.
17. Cornish, HH, and Abar, EL: Toxicity of pyrolysis products of vinyl plastics, Arch Environ Health 19:15, 1969.
18. Curtis, MH, and LeBlanc, PR: 1983 multiple death fires in the United States, Fire J 78:33, 1984.
19. Davies, JWL: Toxic chemicals versus lung tissue—an aspect of inhalation injury revisited, J Burn Care Rehabil 7:213, 1986.
20. Dressler, DP, and Skornik, WA: Effect of antimicrobial therapy on lung bacterial clearance in the burned rat, Ann Surg 175:241, 1972.
21. Dressler, DP, Skornik, WA, and Bloom, SB: Smoke toxicity of commonly available materials, Proceedings of American Industrial Hygiene Association, Minneapolis, Minn., 1975.

22. Dressler, DP, Skornik, WA, and Kupersmith, S: Corticosteroid treatment of experimental smoke inhalation, Ann Surg 183:46, 1976.

23. Dressler, DP, et al: Smoke toxicity of common aircraft carpets, J Aviation, Space, Environ Med 46:1141, 1975.

24. Dressler, DP, et al: Biological effect of fire suppression by nitrogen pressurization in enclosed environments, J Comb Toxicol 4:314, 1977.

25. Durlacher, SH, and Bunting, H: Pulmonary changes following exposure to phosgene, Am J Pathol 23:679, 1947.

26. Dutra, FR: Cerebral residua of acute carbon monoxide poisoning, Am J Clin Pathol 22:925, 1952.

27. Esch, EH, and Dyer, RF: Polyvinyl chloride toxicity in fires: hydrogen chloride toxicity in fire fighters, JAMA 235:393, 1976.

28. Faling, LJ, Medici, TC, and Chodosh, S: Sputum cell population measurements in bronchial injury, Chest 65:56S, 1974.

29. Fechter, LD, and Annau, Z: Toxicity of mild prenatal carbon monoxide exposure, Science 197:680, 1977.

30. Fineberg, C, Miller, BJ, and Allbritten, FF, Jr: Thermal burns of the respiratory tract, Surg Gynecol Obstet 98:318, 1954.

31. Foley, FD, Moncrief, JA, and Mason, AD, Jr: Pathology of the lung in fatally burned patients, Ann Surg 167:251, 1966.

32. Froneberg, BP, Johnson, L, and Landrigan, PJ: Respiratory illness caused by overheating of polyvinyl chloride, Br J Ind Med 39:239, 1982.

33. Garzor, AA: Respiratory mechanics in patients with inhalation burns, J Trauma 10:57, 1970.

34. Getzen, LC, and Pollak, EW: Fatal respiratory distress in burned patients, Surg Gynecol Obstet 152:741, 1981.

35. Henahan, JF: Fire: complicated in America by the ubiquity of plastics, an ancient hazard is becoming even more pernicious, Science 207:29, 1980.

36. Herpol, C: Biological evaluation of the toxicity of products of pyrolysis and combustion of material, Fire Materials 1:29, 1976.

37. Higgins, EA, et al: Acute toxicity of brief exposures to HF, HCL, NO_2, and HCN with and without CO, Fire Technol 8:1200, 1972.

38. Hofman, HTh, and Oettel, H: Comparative toxicity of thermal decomposition products, Mod Plast 46:97, 1969.

39. Hofman, HTh, and Oettel, H: Relative toxicity of thermal decomposition products of expanded polystyrene, J Comb Toxicol 1:236, 1974.

40. Jones, JC: A brief look at the hotel fire record, Fire J 76:38, 1981.

41. Kilmartin, J: Major disaster averted in massive escape of vinyl chloride, Fire J 78:62, 1984.

42. Kimmerle, G: Aspects and methodology for the evaluation of toxicological parameters during fire exposure, J Comb Toxicol 1:4, 1974.

43. Kishitani, K, and Nakamura, K: Toxicities of combustion products, J Fire Flammability & Comb Tox 1:104, 1974.

44. Landa, J, Avery, WG, and Sackner, MA: Some physiological observations in smoke inhalation, Chest 61:62, 1972.

45. Levine, MS, and Radford, EP: Fire victims: medical outcomes and demographic characteristic, Am J Public Health 67:1077, 1977.

46. Liepins, R, and Pearce, EM: Chemistry and toxicity of flame retardants for plastics, Environ Health Perspect 17:55, 1976.

47. Lloyd, EL, and MacRae, WR: Respiratory tract damage in burns: case reports and review of the literature, Br J Anaesth 43:365, 1971.

48. Mallory, TB, and Buckley, WJ: Pathology: with special reference to the pulmonary lesions, Ann Surg 117:865, 1943.

49. McArdle, CS, and Finlay, WEI: Pulmonary complications following smoke inhalation, Br J Anaesth 47:618, 1975.

50. McCord, JM: The superoxide free radical: its biochemistry and pathophysiology, Surgery 94:412, 1983.

51. McFarland, R: Human factors in air transportation, occupational health and safety, New York, 1953, McGraw Hill Book Co.

52. Mellins, RB, and Park, S: Respiratory complications of smoke inhalation in victims of fires, J Pediatr 87:1, 1975.

53. Moritz, AR, and Henriques, FC: Studies of thermal injury. IV. An exploration of the casualty-producing attributes of conflagration: local and systemic effects of general cutaneous exposure to excessive circumambient air and circumradiant heat of varying duration and intensity, Arch Pathol 43:466, 1947.

54. Moritz, AR, Henriques, FC, and McLean, R: Effect of inhaled heat on air passages and lungs, Am J Pathol 21:311, 1945.

55. Moylan, JA: Inhalation injury: a primary de-

terminant of survival following major burns, J Burn Care 2:78, 1981.

56. Moylan, JA, et al: Early diagnosis of inhalation injury using xenon 133 lung scan, Ann Surg 176:477, 1972.

57. Nieman, GF, et al: The effect of smoke inhalation on pulmonary surfactant, Ann Surg 191:171, 1980.

58. Noe, JM, and Constable, JD: A new approach to pulmonary burns: a preliminary report, J Trauma 13:1015, 1973.

59. O'Mara, M: A comparison of combustion products obtained from various synthetic polymers, J Comb Toxicol 1:141, 1974.

60. Oldenburger, D, et al: Inhalation lipoid pneumonia from burning fats: a newly recognized industrial hazard, JAMA 222:1288, 1972.

61. O'Neal, HE, and Benson, SW: Thermochemistry of free radicals in free radicals. Kochi, JK, editor: New York, 1973, John Wiley & Sons.

62. Petajan, JH, et al: Extreme toxicity from combustion products of a fire-retarded polyurethane foam, Science 187:742, 1975.

63. Petroff, PA, et al: Pulmonary function studies after smoke inhalation, Am J Surg 132:346, 1976.

64. Phillips, AW, and Cope, O: Burn therapy. II. The revelation of respiratory tract damage as a principle killer of the burned patient, Ann Surg 155:1, 1962.

65. Phillips, AW, Tanner, JW, and Cope, O: Burn therapy. IV. Respiratory tract damage (an account of the clinical, x-ray and post mortem findings) and the meaning of restlessness, Ann Surg 158:799, 1963.

66. Pietak, SP, and Dlahaye, DJ: Airway obstruction following smoke inhalation, Can Med Assoc J 115:329, 1976.

67. Pruitt, BA, et al: Pulmonary complications in burn patients, J Thorac Cardiovascular Surg 39:7, 1970.

68. Pryor, AJ, Johnson, DE, and Jackson, NN: Hazards of smoke and toxic gases in urban fires, Southwest Research Institute Project 03-2402, Final Report, September 1969.

69. Rapaport, FT, et al: Mechanisms of pulmonary damage in severe burns, Ann Surg 177:472, 1973.

70. Sasaki, J, Cottam, GR, and Baxter, CR: Lipid peroxidation following thermal injury, J Burn Care Rehabil 4:151, 1983.

71. Scheel, LD, Lane, WC, and Coleman, WE: The toxicity of polytetrafluoroethylene pyrolydid products—including carbonyl fluoride and a reaction product, silicon tetrafluoride, Am Ind Hyg Assoc J 29:41, 1968.

72. Scheel, LD, McMillan, L, and Phipps, FC: Biochemical changes associated with toxic exposure to polytetrafluoroethylene pyrolysis products, Am Ind Hyg Assoc J 29:49, 1968.

73. Schwerd, W, and Schulz, E: Carboxyhaemoglobin and methaemoglobin findings in burnt bodies, Forensic Sci Int 12:233, 1978.

74. Shirani, KZ, Pruitt, BA, and Mason, AD, Jr: The influence of inhalation injury and pneumonia on burn mortality, Ann Surg 205:82, 1987.

75. Skornik, WA, Robinson, RS, and Dressler, DP: Toxicity of thermal decomposition products of various paints, J Comb Toxicol 3:71, 1976.

76. Socher, FM, and Mallory, GK: Lung lesions in patients dying of burns, Arch Pathol 75:303, 1983.

77. Stephenson, SF, et al: The pathophysiology of smoke inhalation injury, Ann Surg 182:652, 1975.

78. Stone, HH, and Martin, JD, Jr: Pulmonary injury associated with thermal burns, Surg Gynecol Obstet 129:1242, 1969.

79. Stone, HH, et al: Respiratory burns: a correlation of clinical and laboratory results, Ann Surg 165:157, 1967.

80. Strohl, KP, et al: Carbon monoxide poisoning in fire victims: a reappraisal of prognosis, J Trauma 20:78, 1980.

81. Takahashi, M, et al: Hyperamylasemia in acute carbon monoxide poisoning, J Trauma 22:311, 1982.

82. Taylor, AE, Martin, D, and Parker, JC: The effects of oxygen radicals on pulmonary edema formation, Surgery 94:433, 1983.

83. Taylor, FW, and Gumbert, JL: Cause of death from burns: role of respiratory damage, Ann Surg 161:497, 1965.

84. Terrill, JB, Montgomery, RR, and Reinhardt, CF: Toxic gases from fires, Science 200:1343, 1978.

85. Thorning, DR, et al: Pulmonary responses to smoke inhalation: morphologic changes in rabbits exposed to pine wood smoke, Human Pathol 13:355, 1982.

86. Tse, RL, and Bockman, AA: Nitrogen dioxide toxicity: report of four cases in firemen, JAMA 212:1341, 1970.

87. Tsuchiya, Y, and Sumi, K: Thermal decomposition products of polyvinyl chloride, J Appl Chem 17:364, 1967.

88. United States Navy Flight Surgeons Manual: LC Card 66-61481, 1968, U.S. Government Printing Office.

89. Waritz, RS, and Kwon, BK: The inhalation toxicity of pyrolysis products of polytetrafluoroethylene heated below 500 degrees centigrade, Am Ind Hyg Assoc J 29:19, 1968.

90. Webster, JR, McCabe, MM, and Karp, HF: Recognition and management of smoke inhalation, JAMA 201:287, 1967.

91. Westerberg, LM, Pfaffle, P, and Sundholm, F: Detection of free radicals during processing of polyethylene and polystyrene plastics, Am Ind Hyg Assoc J 43:544, 1982.

92. Wilhelm, DL: Regeneration of tracheal epithelium, J Pathol Bacteriol 65:543, 1953.

93. Wright, PL, and Adams, CH: Toxicity of combustion products from burning polymers: Development and evaluation methods, Environ Health Perspect 17:75, 1976.

94. Zikria, BA, Gerrer, J, and Floch, HF: Wood sawdust vs. kerosene, the chemical factors contributing to pulmonary damage in "Smoke Poisoning," Surgery 71:704, 1972.

95. Zikria, BA, et al: Smoke and carbon monoxide poisoning in fire victims, J Trauma 12:641, 1972.

96. Zikria, BA, et al: What is clinical smoke poisoning? Ann Surg 181:151, 1975.

10 The Minor Burn

DEFINITION OF MINOR BURN

An estimated 200,000 to 300,000 thermally injured patients are admitted to hospitals each year, yet at least 10 times that number are treated and released from emergency departments. Treatment of these patients, at least 3 million people total, has an important impact on patients' health care costs, amount of work missed, abilities to fully function, physical appearances, and most important, comfort.

Although at first it might appear relatively easy to distinguish between minor and major burns, it is always safer to initially diagnose a major injury with subsequent reappraisal than to diagnose a minor injury. This is particularly true in burn care in which the depth and even the extent of the injury frequently cannot be determined for 24 to 48 hours.

A short or overnight admission for evaluation and treatment cannot be criticized by anyone knowledgeable in burn or trauma care. Furthermore this decision should not be challenged by a utilization, diagnosis-related group, or review system. Nevertheless, such a decision can be challenged by patients, their families, and their attorneys.

GUIDELINES FOR AMBULATORY AND HOSPITAL CARE

A minor burn and any concomitant injuries are not by definition life threatening, but admission to a hospital may be appropriate to ensure prompt healing and to improve cosmesis. However, whether a minor burn is treated in the hospital or in an ambulatory setting depends on the specific conditions of the situation.[1,3-6]

Criteria for ambulatory care are as follows:

1. No thermal injury complications, e.g., smoke inhalation
2. Fluid resuscitation completed
3. Stabilized hospital course
4. Adequate nutritional intake
5. Adequate pain tolerance
6. No anticipated septic complications

The psychosocial situation must also be considered when treating a burn patient. Some moderate and even major burns can be treated on an outpatient basis, provided patients satisfactorily meet the medical criteria and family or other members of the household agree to become part of the burn team.

A primary concern in deciding whether a patient can be managed on an ambulatory basis is an assessment of whether he or she is able and can be trusted to follow instructions (i.e., "patient compliance") such as those provided below in the following list:

1. Bathe the wound twice daily with warm water and mild soap, soaking off the dressing if necessary. Rinse thoroughly and then apply dressing as necessary, depending on location and age of burn. Shower, but do not bathe in a bathtub unless perineum is burned.
2. Call or return if pain, fever, redness, and/or pus persist.
3. Return to clinic by appointment or by request of patient, health care provider, or even social workers if patient is failing to meet appointments.

These instructions should be written and reviewed with the patient and/or his family. If the patient is an outpatient, a follow-up visit by either the visiting nurse or treating physician is mandatory within 24 hours and thereafter as required.

The burn wound criteria for hospital admission are as follows:

1. More than 5% BSA second- and third-degree burn
2. Third-degree burn more than 2% BSA
3. Patients younger than age 5 or older than age 60
4. Airway, inhalation, or electrical injury
5. Significant associate injury or preexisting disease
6. Deep burns of face, hands, feet, or perineum
7. Suspected child abuse
8. Presence of other illnesses or injuries

These criteria apply to major burns as well as minor ones. Even though some patients with minor burns should be admitted to a hospital, it is unusual to treat a major burn on an ambulatory care basis. Therefore these guidelines are primarily to evaluate patients with minor burns, particularly those with full-thickness burns amendable to primary excision.

A treatment protocol for minor burns is as follows:
1. Evaluate burn
2. Evaluate other injuries or diseases
3. Apply cold/ice water compresses to area of burn
4. Wash wound thoroughly with dilute chlorhexidine gluconate (Hibiclens) (30 ml/L)
5. Apply dry, sterile dressing
6. Give tetanus booster as needed if no immunization within 5 years, add human tetanus immune globulin (Hypertet) if no immunization record
7. Complete history and physical record, including burn size and depth description and associated complicating factors
8. Administer analgesic, systemic or oral, determined by patient's age and size
9. Instruct patient and family (bilingually, if necessary)

The same general principles apply to the minor burn as the major burn, but one difference is that the minor burn usually has no systemic effects. The minor burn wound retains a barrier to invasive sepsis. However, this is not the case with small third-degree burns treated on an ambulatory basis. The same topical care is needed to prevent infection in these small burns as in larger burns. Cosmetic and functional results, which are also often overlooked in caring for the minor burn, must be fully considered.

Another example of the similarity in care for both minor and major burns is that both require reducing the accumulation of exudate, necrotic tissue, and the number of bacteria at the wound site so as to reduce the probability of invasive wound sepsis. This is done either by leaving the burn wound uncovered or with as little protective dressing as necessary to prevent chaffing. Frequent washing is also a part of treatment, although it is often difficult to convince the patient that it is advantageous to wash the injured area. Active and passive motion early in the process is also encouraged to reduce the possibility of loss of function and to contribute to the patient's overall well-being.

COMMON PROBLEMS

In treating a minor and, in most cases, an ambulatory burn, discussing common problems in both cause and treatment of these burns will help clarify procedures.

Sunburn

Sunburns happen almost as frequently as minor kitchen burns. They are preventable with proper use of sunscreens. A sunburn can be extensive; it can be both second degree and first degree. Third-degree burns rarely occur, except in particularly sensitive children, and they rarely convert to third-degree even with sepsis. The same guidelines pertain to sunburns as to all other burns. Primarily because of the cause of sunburns people have a tendency to downgrade their importance. Although most sunburn occurs in young, healthy adults or older children and not in the elderly or infants, the latter are particularly susceptible. The importance of treating sunburns in these patients cannot be overstressed.

In youthful patients it is often very difficult to determine initially both the depth and percent of total BSA involved. Therefore it is prudent to lean heavily toward admitting these children for at least 24 to 72 hours for an injury that in adults would be considered a minor burn. In youthful cases hyperthermia and hypovolemia with shock, sepsis, and possibly deeper burn injury and its effects may occur. Treatment is observation, analgesics, and intravenous fluids, as well as appropriate burn wound care.

In the ambulatory patient with a minor sunburn, treatment is similar to that for other minor burns, except that the first-degree area can be extensive and require analgesics or even intravenous fluids. The patient should be admitted to a hospital if he is very uncomfortable, nauseated, or has other extenuating medical or social problems.

In the management of these extensive sunburns pains and chills are the two most frequent problems. During the first 24 hours patients often have severe pain that cannot be controlled by prolonged application of ice or cold compresses. In this case parenteral narcotics are often the only effective therapy. Small frequent doses are desirable as in any injury, but dosage may be difficult to control if the patient is not hospitalized. To provide immediate pain relief and continued analgesia at home, a combination of parenteral and oral medication is often given in dosages that correlate with the drugs' varying absorption rates and durations.

Although patients in their homes may require considerable medication, it is easy to be lured into giving high doses to prolong the effect rather than developing a protocol for administering smaller parenteral doses that may be more acceptable, particularly when acute pain and accompanying anxiety are relieved. Thereafter a combination of parenteral and oral analgesics usually suffice. If it is necessary, a brief overnight hospital stay may be best for the patient and greatly facilitate patient acceptance, compliance, satisfaction, and earlier return to full activity.

Fortuitously, parenteral or oral medication absorption in sunburn patients is not a problem unless the patient has other mitigating diseases; care must be taken with the diabetic patient or the elderly patient with peripheral vascular disease.

Patients with extensive sunburn frequently develop severe shaking chills of the type often seen with acute bacteremia. This usually occurs during the 12- to 36-hour postburn period and is probably caused by fluid loss that, in turn, is caused by capillary permeability and obligatory water loss aggravated by anxiety and abundant application of cold water therapy. After first eliminating the possibility of sepsis, treatment is to replace fluid losses orally, if feasible, with warm liquids. It is important to include sedatives in addition to analgesics, since the problem is often anxiety coupled with pain.

A summary of the treatment of sunburn follows:

1. General evaluation, i.e., history, physical examination, and laboratory tests as indicated
2. Cool and wet compresses on burn wound as long as acute pain persists, sometimes hours
3. Systemic, oral, or parenteral analgesic and/or sedative
4. Topical medication if indicated, see following section
5. Dressings only in selected high-exposure areas
6. No antibiotics unless treating an actual infection
7. Tetanus immunization if indicated

Topical creams, ointments, emollients, and sprays

In first-degree burns the skin retains its normal functions such as acting as a barrier to infection and absorbing chemicals (i.e., medications). Many minor burns, however, contain some second-degree areas where sepsis is possible or where absorption of medication could cause allergic reaction. Therefore correct diagnosis of the depth and degree of the burn, a thorough allergy history, and adherence, first to the principles that govern absorption of medication through the skin, and second to the purpose of the application are of primary importance.

Absorption. All substances or agents possess the potential for absorption. Specifically, absorption depends on the vehicle (i.e., water or oil base), an agent's release rate, solubility, concentration in the topical vehicle, and the size of the molecule. The presence of a water-to-water interface between the skin and the topical agent and vehicle is critical, as is the thickness of the skin and eschar. Eschar, even eschar that appears dry, is not a barrier to absorption, insensible water loss, or invasion of bacteria.

Therefore agents in a cream- or water-based vehicle will absorb at a faster rate as long as the vehicle or cream maintains its moisture. In an uncovered wound absorption time is usually less than 30 minutes following application. Conversely, agents in an oil or petrolatum ointment base are released and absorbed at a much slower rate, but they may be applied for a much longer period of time. Ointments, however, do not easily wash off a wound and may in effect seal a wound, thereby increasing the possibility of maceration and sepsis.

Analgesia. In a minor burn systemic analgesics are not frequent, and absorption and possible toxicity from the analgesic agent is not a problem. Following or supplementing application of cold or ice water, several commercially available products containing 9.4% benzocaine or 2 to 2.5% lidocaine are effective. They may need to be supplemented with a systemic analgesic or sedative for the first day or so.

Cleaning of eschar, foreign material, and bacteria. Cleansing the wound is essential. Although this process should begin as soon as possible, it is not necessary to start before the patient is evaluated and given relief for pain. Then a gentle washing with an antiseptic and rinsing are desirable. It is important to repeat the washing process at least twice a day until the wound is healed. Obviously, a wound sealed with an oil- or petrolatum-based ointment cannot be easily washed or cleaned. Abundant warm water at a temperature most comfortable for the patient is best. Usually the water is tepid at first and fairly warm later. Sterile water is not necessary, but good cleaning technique is important. Hydrogen peroxide diluted to 1.5% (half of the commercially available 3%) may be useful to dissolve exudate and blood clots, but it only has secondary or indirect antiseptic value.

Prevention or treatment of sepsis. Again, if the burn is only first degree, infection is hardly a risk. However, the wound often has second-degree areas that have temporary loss of barrier function as indicated by edema, blisters, and exudate. At the very least, there is always one bacterium even if the host resistance condition (i.e., the injured skin and milieu) is strong.

Therefore it is always prudent to recognize the probability of bacterial contamination and the possibility of infection. Although minor burns are not usually susceptible to infection, it is possible for a second-degree burn to be converted to a third-degree injury because of sepsis, wound pressure, or maceration. This thereby increases the possibility of grafting, cosmetic or functional deformity, and, minimally, delay in wound healing.

The best prevention and, if necessary, treatment of invasive sepsis is a clean wound adequately protected against further injury. Topical antimicrobials, silver sulfadiazine, or mafenide are not usually used on a minor wound. However, an exception should be made if the location is particularly susceptible (e.g., perineum), since burns in these areas should not be considered minor wounds.

The use of topical antiinfectives like povidone-iodine (Betadine) and nitrofurazone have not been shown to have any greater value than regular clean wound care. However, they are commercially available in an excellent water-soluble cream and therefore are washed off easily and permit thorough cleaning of the wound. In addition, use of a dressing will reduce bacterial growth in the exudate that collects in the interstices of the dressing. The exact benefit of this is not clear, since a first-degree burn wound, by definition, retains its barrier function. However, although the principle is sound, as previously discussed, some areas in a minor burn are often susceptible to second-degree injury.

Allergy rates must be considered with most of these agents. This has been shown to be 9.5% with prolonged use of Sulfamylon and 5% with nitrofurazone. Obviously, the same precautions should be taken with these agents as with any other medications to avoid allergic reactions. Fortunately, their use for treatment of minor burns is helpful, but not critical.

Protection of the wound. Some wounds need a dressing for protection. Topical treatments do not protect a wound. In the past and even today some aerosol plastic sprays have been applied. These sprays offer no analgesic effect and may macerate a wound because of increased insensible water loss and sweating. If the wound has any second-degree areas, bacteria that cannot be completely removed may result in invasive burn wound sepsis. If the dressing may adhere to the wound, a small amount of a cream- or water-based vehicle may be applied. In actual practice, however, adherence is not a problem because the dressing can be soaked or washed off. Given a little time to rehydrate, a dressing that adheres will provide gentle and effective debridement.

Psychologic pressure. Psychologic pressure motivates people to cover the burn wound with some type of cream or ointment. Traditionally, the soothing effect of the application of some topical treatments is not entirely psychologic, although it would be difficult to prove this statistically. Like the patient, the health-care provider may equate an open, bare wound with an untreated wound. As long as the basic principles of wound care are observed, applying these materials to a minor first-degree burn is harmless. If a "cover-up" must be used, use something that washes off readily in the daily washes, is not highly allergenic, has low absorption and toxicity levels, and costs a minimum amount.

Debridement of bullae

Several common examples of second-degree burns with extensive bullae development are shown in Figs. 10-1 and 10-2. Fig. 10-1 shows a relatively minor second-degree burn on the ankle that can easily infect and convert to third degree. Although this wound would not usually be disabling on a permanent basis, its location interferes with wearing shoes and therefore makes it difficult to return to work.

In contrast, the hand burn shown in Fig. 10-2 can lead to a permanent disability if not properly treated. It is difficult to make a decision about whether or not to debride these bullae. Although early removal prevents exudate rich in bacterial nutrients, retention of the bullae is often more comfortable. The bullae prevent the wound from drying out, causing patient discomfort and injury to any remaining viable epithelial cells. They also provide a temporary barrier to invasive bacteria.

Recommended treatment is careful cleansing of the wound followed by application of a topical antimicrobial agent and preservation of the intact bullae. If the bullae have been ruptured but are otherwise intact, it is recommended that they be retained in place for at least several days, with care being taken to cleanse carefully and to debride earlier than otherwise indicated. In any case, the wound must be inspected at least every day, and the bullae must be completely debrided at the earliest sign of any cloudy collection or erythema. The wound and fluid should be cultured, and the newly exposed wound treated promptly with an antibacterial agent. The bullae usually break during the cleansing process or accidentally from pressure around the fifth to the seventh day. If the wound can be kept free from bacterial invasion, removal of the bullae would expose a second-degree wound with thin but pink, healing epithelium.

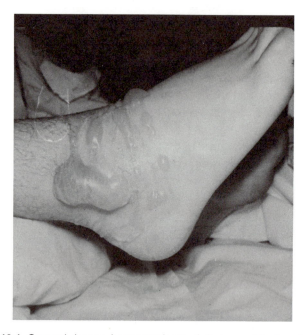

Fig. 10-1. Second-degree hot water burn of dorsum of foot and ankle.

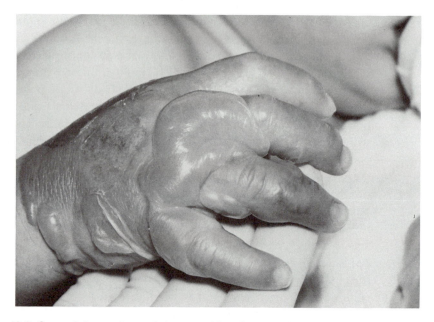

Fig. 10-2. Second-degree burn of dorsum of hand caused by hot water in child with large bullae.

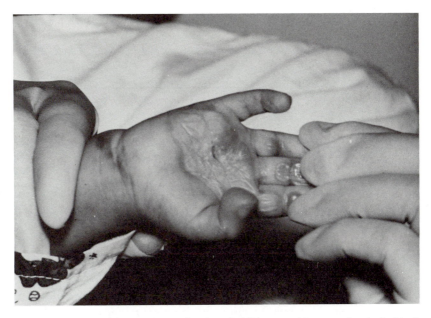

Fig. 10-3. Second-degree burn of palm of child caused by grasping hot object.

Hand burns

Hands are one of the most common areas of minor burn. Inadequate treatment that results in extensive inflammatory reaction or development of invasive burn wound sepsis, no matter how minor, can result in scarring and severe dysfunction. Fig. 10-3 shows a second-degree burn in the palm of a child who grasped a hot object. This is a relatively common minor burn. Even though the best treatment is always prevention, these burns are treated most effectively by frequent washing and soaking with an antiseptic agent and encouraging the child to play and use the hand actively and passively. This will help prevent sepsis and inflammation of the tendon sheaths and joint capsules. Because of the thickness of the palm, this injury rarely requires grafting.

Socioeconomic issues

Socioeconomic issues are a very real problem in caring for the patient with a minor burn. These problems can range from possible child abuse or neglect to arranging supportive or nursing care for the elderly. Frequently, patients need to be admitted to a hospital for a short time until such care or support can be provided. Immediate involvement of public and private authorities and/or agencies is a legal requirement in most jurisdictions. Although the procedure may often encounter resistance from house staff, administrators, and insurance carriers, it (i.e., extended protection of the patient) will probably save unnecessary expenditure, including legal expense, and, of course, reduce morbidity.

DRESSINGS
What to use

To function properly a dressing must consist of three functional layers: a contact layer, an absorbent layer, and a protective layer. In practice these layers can be combined.

The contact layer is placed next to the wound. This layer is sometimes impregnated with a therapeutic agent such as an antimicrobial agent in a vehicle or more commonly just a vehicle such as petrolatum or vaseline. Although the optimum material should permit access for drainage, the use of plastic such as Telfa, which has nonadherent properties, is very common. Regrettably, these materials do not readily permit drainage of the exudate, and thus they provide an excellent media for bacterial growth and maceration. The nonadherent quality is based on the nonadherence of pus, which is easily observable on the removed dressing. Plain gauze made of a not too fine mesh will adhere to a wound, but gently removing it with water will also provide some beneficial debridement.

The absorbent layer should be thick enough to absorb all the exudate expected to accumulate within a reasonable period of time. Ideally it also provides some protection by cushioning the wound by distributing pressure. Some absorbent layers contain antimicrobial agents that act primarily to prevent bacteria from growing in the interstices of the dressing, but these are of doubtful value, since the dressing should be changed when the layer is saturated.

The outer protective layer not only protects the wound from external trauma, but also prevents leakage of the wound exudate or drainage fluids. It should be occlusive and, like all materials in a dressing, sterilized with a long shelf life. Obviously no matter how hygienically packaged or aerosolized, single-layer plastic materials will result in exudate pooling, which is always contaminated with bacteria and promotes maceration and sepsis.

When to change dressings

Dressings should be changed for the following reasons: examination of the wound, debridement and/or closure, and prevention of maceration and sepsis because of collection of drainage fluid. In the minor burn patient the dressing should be changed, and the wound examined 24 hours after its application. This is especially pertinent in a thermal wound patient because of the inherent difficulty in evaluating the fresh burn wound. Thereafter the dressing is best changed at least daily and accompanied by gentle cleansing and debridement if necessary. Depending on the circumstances, this treatment could be performed by the family, visiting nurse, physician, or the patient himself. At this time only fibrin and not tissue will have become enmeshed in the contact layer. Therefore removal of the dressing should not be very uncomfortable.

If the dressing remains unchanged for 3 to 4 days and is not septic, an open wound will have ingrowth of granulation tissue, and removal of the dressing will cause some pain. As in all burn cases, it is important to examine the used dressing for signs of sepsis.

COMMON COMPLICATIONS
Sepsis

Sepsis is undoubtedly the most common complication following a minor burn. Most of these infections are superficial and not invasive. Sepsis can be easily diagnosed by examining the dressing for purulent exudate. The organisms are most often staphylococci. As long as sepsis has not invaded the wound, it should be washed frequently and either be left to air dry or covered by a plain gauze dressing. If bacterial invasion develops as indicated by local cellulitis, regional lymphangitis and lymphadenopathy, or systemic signs or symptoms, both topical and parenteral antibiotics should be given. Since the common organism in these cases of bacterial invasion is streptococcus, penicillin is commonly given. On occasion the patient should be hospitalized until the burn wound sepsis is controlled.

Misjudgment of depth and percent of area burned

The percent of area burned is frequently misjudged, but this is rarely a problem unless the patient is a child. In these cases the rule of nines should be applied. For example, if a child has been burned on the side of the face, neck, and shoulder from pulling a container of hot liquid off a table, he or she may be diagnosed as having a minor 5% to 7% BSA burn, whereas in reality the injury is major (i.e., 12% to 15% BSA). Misjudgment of burn wound depth is frequent, particularly when distinguishing deep second-degree burns from third-degree ones. However, it is also not uncommon to convert a second-degree burn to third degree because of sepsis and maceration without ever recognizing that the wound was initially a second-degree injury. It is also exceedingly difficult to diagnose depth very early in the postburn period unless the burn is either clearly first or third degree.[2]

Allergic reaction to medication

Allergic reactions have been reported in 9.5% of 400 patients treated for an average of 26 days with Sulfamylon.[1] Of the reactions, 39 were local reactions manifested by erythema and urticaria. Although these reactions usually respond readily to antihistamines, two cases of erythema multiforme were reported. Since effective medication alternatives are available, it is recommended that these patients be changed to another agent.[7]

Allergic reactions to sulfadiazine silver have not been reported. Application of nitrofurazone results in a 5% incidence of local dermatitis. Other allergic reactions such as reaction to penicillin can also occur and can confuse the appearance of the burn wound.

Delayed healing

Delayed healing of a minor burn is usually caused either by sepsis or misjudgment of the burn depth. A burn in areas exposed to trauma, body fluid, or moisture can also result in maceration and delayed healing. Other problems to be alert for are diabetes mellitus, peripheral vascular disease, collagen diseases, or any disease that results in edema or metabolic imbalance, including malnutrition.

Persistent hyperpigmentation or hypopigmentation

Persistent hyperpigmentation or hypopigmentation of the area of a minor burn can be a problem. Considerable reassurance of the patient is often necessary. Overall, surgery has not been very beneficial in this domain. Fading of the pigmented areas occurs over time, even several years. It is not uncommon, however, to have only patchy repigmentation. In such cases, particularly if a large area of the face is involved, serious social and psychologic problems can require psychotherapy.

Scarring

Scarring is rarely a problem with a minor burn unless cosmesis or hand functioning is involved. Poor quality skin can result from the reepithelization of deep second-degree burns because of the body's failure to restructure the normal dermis. Problems can arise because of the poor quality of the skin and its tendency to break down, ulcerate, and become septic. Customary treatment is to protect and support the skin with topical emollients. Surgery is rarely required. A healing time of 6 months to a year is to be expected.

SUMMARY

The minor burn is one of the most common and most neglected injuries. The approach that all will heal regardless of treatment or depending on individual physician idiosyncrasies leads to much discomfort, poor results, and, most important, patient dissatisfaction.

It is imperative to keep principles of burn wound care at the forefront in treating the minor burn. With increasing emphasis on ambulatory care and the general improvement in home health care, educating and training health care providers and the public to keep up with the emerging trends in caring for thermally injured patients is a challenge.

REFERENCES

1. Bruck, HM: The management of small burns. In Artz, CP, Moncrief, JA, and Pruitt, BA, editors: Burns: a team approach, Philadelphia, 1979, WB Saunders Co.
2. Hinshaw, JR, and Payne, FW: The restoration and remodeling of the skin after a second degree burn, Surg Gynecol Obstet 117:738, 1963.
3. Miller, SF, Finley, RK, and Alkire, S: The management of small full-thickness burns by primary excision, J Burn Care 1:10, 1980.
4. Nance, FC, et al: Aggressive outpatient care of burns, J Trauma 12:144, 1972.
5. O'Neil, JA: Burns—office evaluation and management, Primary Care 3:531, 1976.
6. Warden, G, Kravitz, M, and Schnebly, A: The outpatient management of moderate and major thermal injuries, J Burn Care 2:159, 1981.
7. Yaffee, HS, and Dressler, DP: Topical application of mafenide acetate: its association with erythema multiforme and cutaneous reactions, Arch Dermatol 100:277, 1969.

11 Treatment Problems

OVERVIEW

A number of clinical problems are frequently encountered and somewhat unique to the treatment of the thermally injured patient. They fall into several categories such as fluid therapy or constriction of the thoracic cage or an extremity because of swelling of a circumferential burn, hypertension, development of Curling's ulcer, hypothermia, or idiopathic diabetes.

Recognition and treatment of these problems depend on thorough knowledge of critical care pathophysiology, of all facets of burn injury, and of the often adverse effects of therapy. With these foundations, finding solutions is most easily approached from a checklist basis.

PEDIATRIC PROBLEMS

Mortality and morbidity in groups of patients over the age of 65 and younger than age 5 are significantly increased. The many reasons for this include the different circumstances in which these patients are injured. Some of the other contributing factors are considered in the following section.[4,6,12,13]

Estimation of burn depth and size

Children have a higher ratio of BSA to weight than adults. Thus their fluid loss may be higher than current fluid formula charts indicate. Wide fluctuation of body temperature may also occur and alter fluid needs. Therefore constant reassessment is necessary.

The severity of scald burns, the most common injury in children, is often underestimated. In 1947 Moritz and Henriques[17] showed that the time required to produce a full-thickness burn on human cadaver was less than 5 seconds in water with a mean temperature of 130° F (54° C) and 10 minutes in water with a mean temperature of 120° F (49° C). This time was shorter in children.

A review of the Lund-Browder chart (see Fig. 3-1) for children shows that a newborn's head and neck represents 19% of BSA whereas this area is 9% in an adult. A lack of recognition of this fact leads to inappropriate care.

Fig. 11-1 shows second- and third-degree burns of a child's face, ear, neck, shoulder, and anterior trunk caused by spilling a hot liquid. This accident commonly occurs when a child reaches up and pulls a container of hot liquid, usually water or soup, off a table or stove. Because of variation in distribution of BSA between adults and children, this type of burn is often misclassified as a minor burn (i.e., less than 10% total BSA second-degree burn in an adult). In reality, it is a burn over 15% total BSA in a 2-year-old patient. Thus the patient should be admitted for at least 24 hours until the depth of the burn is determined. Exposure to the same heat for the same amount of time that would cause a partial-thickness injury in an adult is more apt to cause a third-degree burn on the thin skin of a child.

Fluid management

Children less than age 3 need a urine output level of 2 to 2.5 ml/kg/hour to assure adequate perfusion of the kidneys, vs. 0.5 to 1.5 ml/kg/hour in older children. Therefore to err slightly by giving too much fluid to children is desirable, especially since their young and presumed healthy cardiovascular system has less chance of creating a fluid overload.

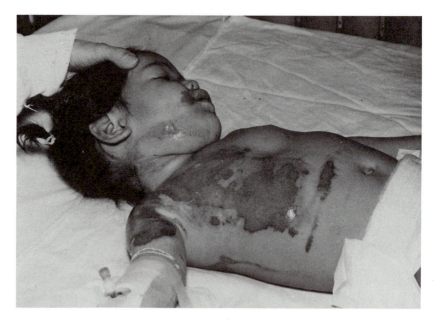

Fig. 11-1. Second- and third-degree burn in child resulting in 15% total BSA burn caused by hot liquid.

Table 11-1. Effect of edema on airway cross-sectional area

Tracheal diameter (mm)	Cross-sectional area (mm²)	Cross-sectional area with 1 mm edema (mm²)	Reduction (%)
14	153	113	26
6	28	12.6	55

Respiratory support

Since resistance to flow is equal to the diameter of the airway to the fourth power, a small reduction in diameter because of edema can be much more disastrous in a child than in an adult. Table 11-1 shows the effect of edema on a cross-sectional area of the airway in a typical adult and child. Failure to realize this can cause inadequate ventilation.

Dosage differences

Caring for the burned child requires distinct differences in dosages, mainly in analgesics and antimicrobials. It is not uncommon to find the pediatric patient undermedicated. Similar to adults, children need to have the medication titrated. On the other hand, children are often overmedicated with both topical and systemic antimicrobial agents, which causes an increase in the incidence and severity of side effects.

Psychiatric aspects

In addition to the immediate psychiatric effects on the burned child, the long-term effects not only on the patient but on family and friends are often not fully appreciated. Although these effects will not be discussed here, the need for early involvement of a qualified professional in this area is apparent.

Child abuse

A burned child must always raise suspicions about parental or guardian abuse. The abuse pattern most common is immersion into a tub or sink that results in scalding of the buttocks, perineum, or legs. However, a diagnosis of child abuse is often confused with neglect or accident. It is most important to handle the subject or suspicion tactfully but thoroughly. Hasty accusations can lead to lasting psychiatric problems in addition to legal liability.[3,10]

Various indices of possible child abuse are as follows:
1. History of repeated injuries, delays in seeking care
2. Discrepancies in explanations of injuries or in history and nature of injuries
3. Injuries found in physical examination and x-ray films not reported by parents
4. General nutrition and health poor
5. Child extremely passive, compliant, or fearful
6. Evidence of sexual activity or abuse
7. Bruises or broken bones in an infant younger than 12 months old
8. X-ray films showing a chip or metaphysical fracture in joints (a result of twisted limbs)
9. Head injuries
10. Abdominal or internal injuries
11. Behavior of parents: overreact or underreact, cannot remember how it happened, insensitive to child's pain or condition, refuse consent for further examination of child, blame others, appear detached or apathetic
12. "Hospital shoppers": those people who for no apparent reason have brought an injured child to a hospital outside their community when their own community has fully equipped facilities

Note that these are only "suspicions" and indicate the need for further investigation.

Fig. 11-2 shows a second-degree burn of the buttocks and feet highly suggestive of a child abuse injury. This injury occurs when a child is lowered into a container of

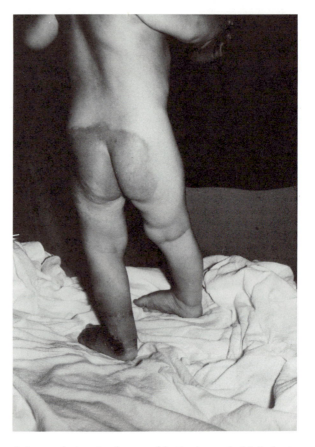

Fig. 11-2. Second-degree hot water burns of buttocks and child's feet caused by abuse.

hot water. Because the child is held by his arms, his feet are drawn up so that his ankles but not usually his toes are burned. On the other hand, if the child stepped into a tub of water that is too hot, only his feet and not his buttocks would be burned. Even considering possible variations in water temperature and the higher susceptibility of the buttocks to burn injury vs. the relatively thick skin of the feet, the feet would still have a more severe burn injury. Whether the child is lowered accidentally or on purpose (i.e., out of neglect or abuse), the issue still needs to be investigated by appropriate authorities.

GERIATRIC DIFFICULTIES

Not only is the mortality rate increased in the burned geriatric patient, but differences in rehabilitation have profound effects. Among the factors adversely affecting these patients are the following[1,2,4,16]:

1. Multiple diseases and medications
2. Multiple health care providers
3. Decreased water percentage (i.e., 61% to 53% water volume) and an increased fat percentage, from 14% to 21%, that complicates fluid resuscitation
4. Decreased renal and hepatic functioning that could make a significant impact on medication absorption, concentration, metabolism, and excretion
5. Increased opportunity for and percent of adverse drug interactions
6. Possible unreliability of renal functioning as measured by creatinine clearance
7. Possible confusion caused by cimetidine given in normal doses of 300 mg q.i.d.
8. Prescribed medication not taken because of confusion or cost
9. Presumption of presence of cardiopulmonary diseases and anticipation of complications, so common in this age group

CIRCUMFERENTIAL BURNS

A circumferential burn of the limbs or thoracic cage can cause compression of the vascular system and loss of pulmonary compliance because of rapidly accumulating edema. This usually takes several hours to develop, but the effect can cause ventilatory distress while the patient is still in the emergency room. As the edema fluid increases in the burn wound and subcutaneous tissue, the burn skin has a diminished ability to accommodate by stretching. If the burn encompasses an extremity or the thoracic cage, compression and compromise of the underlying tissue structures or decreased pulmonary compliance can result. A deeper third- or fourth-degree burn has less ability to expand and is more apt to decrease pulmonary compliance. This rapidly subsides, generally between 48 and 72 hours postburn. Yet a burn that is not quite fully circumferential may be unable to allow for the massive edema, and escharotomy should be considered. Prompt recognition and treatment can save both life and limb.

Indications for escharotomy

Indications for escharotomy in treating constricting circumferential burns are:
1. Circumferential burn
2. Decreased compliance and respiratory function
3. Signs of decreased peripheral circulation

Escharotomy is incision into burn eschar to relieve the constricting effect and allow the underlying tissue to expand because of edema. Timely performance of escharotomy can save a vascularly compromised limb or a life by releasing the constricting effect of a circumferential third-degree burn on pulmonary functioning. Although this swelling and constriction can occur within a few minutes following a burn injury, this is rarely the case. It is unusual for these indications to be evident while the patient is in the emergency room, except if he or she has a very severe and extensive chest burn. The usual time for occurrence of these indications is from 6 to 18 hours postburn when the edema has peaked if the patient has been properly managed. Thus the edema and concomitant constriction start to subside.

Decreased compliance and respiratory function. The need for an escharotomy is often identified by the increasing difficulty in ventilating the patient because of decreased compliance. Further confirmation of the positive results of a chest-wall escharotomy is shown in the immediate improvement in respiratory function.

Signs of decreased peripheral circulation. Monitoring various pulses and recording results is the easiest method of assessing the need for an escharotomy. Unfortunately, the developing edema may make this method unreliable. Similarly, clinical evaluation of peripheral perfusion by Doppler scanning or examination of the function, color, or refill of the nailbeds can also be difficult and reflect other reasons for diminished perfusion. In these instances it is safer to make a diagnosis based on an assessment of the burn wound and the results of an escharotomy.

Pain. Pain may be an acute sign early in the course in vascularly compromised extremities, but this lessens gradually as the complications progress. Pain may be masked by analgesics so that pain in itself is an unreliable finding in indicating the need for an escharotomy.

Technique for escharotomy

Fig. 11-3 shows an escharotomy site on the lateral aspect of the lower extremity of a pediatric patient. This wound is 7 days old and demonstrates the bulging nature of the subcutaneous tissue at first caused by edema and then by granulation tissue. In those cases properly selected for escharotomy, the incision will not cause any additional deformity or delay in healing, since the adjacent area is already fully involved. Technique for escharotomy is as follows:

1. Keep everything sterile
2. Incise full thickness of burn or eschar
3. Control bleeding
4. Treat newly opened wounds with topical antimicrobial therapy
5. Monitor results

Sterile technique. Every attempt should be made not to further contaminate the burn wound. Sterile technique, including masks, gowns, gloves, drapes, and wound preparations will reduce the inoculum.

Incision of full-thickness of burn or eschar. An incision is made through full-thickness of burn or eschar. This should result in a bulging of the edematous, subcutaneous tissue that should be bloodless. The incision must extend slightly above and below the burned, constricted area for maximum effect. Like all incisions, it should not be placed across joints so as not to adversely affect motion. Usually, an incision is made on both sides on an extremity or the chest wall, either along the

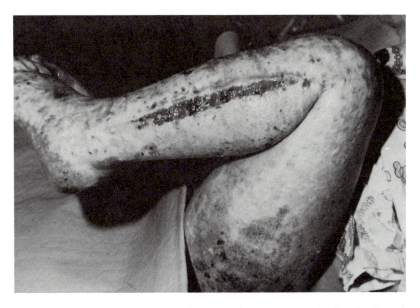

Fig. 11-3. Escharotomy incision on lateral aspect of lower extremity of pediatric patient at 7 days.

slightly anterolateral margin of the chest or medially and laterally along the extremity.

Occasionally, inexperienced personnel, in their enthusiasm, will incise too deeply (i.e., beneath the burn eschar) into viable tissue. This is best prevented by the supervision of experienced and qualified staff. However, if this occurs, the wound must be repaired similar to any other laceration, except for one step. Since the wound contains nonviable tissue in the form of eschar, it must be left open to heal by secondary or tertiary intention.

Control of bleeding. Even with optimum conditions, bleeding from the escharotomy site can be a problem. The more severe the burn, the less the possibility of this complication. Care must be taken to only incise to the proper depth. Treatment is ligation of the bleeders, usually done most easily with suture ligatures because of the extreme friability of the burned tissue, application of hemostatic agents such as fibrin or thrombin, and pressure.

Treatment of open wound with antimicrobials. In an effort to control bleeding or in failure to recognize the escharotomy site as an open, bacterially contaminated extension of the adjacent burn wound, escharotomy wounds are often treated differently from other burn injuries. These wounds should be treated uncovered and with the same cleansing procedures and topical antimicrobial agents as other burn wounds.

Monitoring of results. If the escharotomy is successful, immediate improvement in perfusion of an extremity and even a lessening of pain will usually occur. Releasing constriction of the thoracic cage can be even more dramatic, showing a rapid improvement in breathing pattern, clinical signs, and blood gases. These events usually occur within a few minutes, but the patient will show a more gradual improvement during the 1 to 2 hours after escharotomy. If the patient shows no immediate improvement, the wound must be reexamined for the adequacy of the escharotomy, the possibility of other causes of diminished peripheral perfusion, or pulmonary compliance.

OTHER PROBLEMS
Hypertension

Frequency. Hypertension is a common complication in major burns. All patients with severe burns should have their blood pressures recorded at least four times a day, and patients who maintain a diastolic blood pressure of 100 torr during two readings 30 minutes apart require treatment. Hydralazine is the drug usually used. Recommended dosages are identified below. However, the patient may need improved respiratory support, correction of pH and blood gas abnormalities, sedation, or analgesia.[8,18]

Diagnosis. Once the aforementioned causes for hypertension are excluded, the diagnosis is straightforward. The patient can be monitored by blood pressure readings to determine the efficacy of treatment and to be certain that the diagnosis is correct.

Treatment. Recommended dosages for hydralazine are as follows:

1. Intramuscular hydralazine: A 0.15 mg/kg dose may be repeated every 6 to 12 hours. After a course is initiated, hydralazine should be continued for at least 3 days, unless diastolic blood pressure falls below 80.
2. Oral hydralazine: This is generally not recommended in a critical situation.
3. The aim is to keep the diastolic pressure below 100 torr. The dose of hydralazine should be increased until this has occurred or undesirable side effects have developed.
4. In the event that satisfactory control of the pressure cannot be secured by use of hydralazine, another drug may be used, usually methyldopa.
5. Methyldopa:
   a. Children receive 5 to 10 mg/kg every 6 hours IV in 100 ml of 5% glucose over 30 minutes.
   b. Adults receive 250 mg every 6 hours IV in 100 ml dextrose.

Curling's ulcer

Incidence and prevention. Stress ulcers (Curling's ulcer) used to be frequent sequelae of extensive burns. With the improved nutritional support available in the past 10 to 15 years through parenteral routes, the incidence of ulceration and bleeding from the upper gastrointestinal tract has decreased. Past experience has shown a close association between invasive burn wound sepsis and upper gastrointestinal bleeding. Patients who are septic should be treated prophylactically with antacids and cimetidine.

When the patient is on a regular diet with interval feedings, the resultant hyperacidity can be controlled, and erosions and ulcerations of the upper gastrointestinal tract are rare. If a normal oral intake cannot be taken, all patients with moderate or large burns should be started on antacid therapy. The antacid therapy of choice is either aluminum hydroxide gel (Amphogel) or magnesium hydroxide-aluminum hydroxide (Mylanta).

Conservative treatment. A bleeding profile should be obtained to eliminate disseminated intravascular coagulation as a possible cause of upper gastrointestinal bleeding. If any of the clotting factors are in question, fresh frozen plasma should be infused with packed red cells to return blood volume to normal. When cimetidine, packed red cells, fresh frozen plasma, and antacids have been instituted and continued for a period of 10 to 15 days, many erosions or early ulcerations will heal without surgical intervention.

Irrigation of the stomach with ice water has not been helpful in controlling bleeding. Important adjunctive treatments during this critical period include precise control of local and invasive burn wound infections and aggressive closure of the wound.

Cimetidine, a histamine H_2-receptor antagonist, may also be used in patients who have extensive burns complicated by invasive sepsis. Not an anticholinergic agent, cimetidine blocks histamine-stimulated gastric acid secretion by parietal cells and may also decrease gastric edema. It also inhibits gastric acid secretion stimulated by insulin, pentagastrin, food, or physiologic vagal reflex. A single 300-mg tablet taken orally in a clinical setting raises intragastric pH to 5 and inhibits basal gastric acid secretion by 100% for at least 2 hours. Inhibition is still 90% after 4 hours. However, stimulated acid secretion is 50% inhibited, pentagastrin 60%, insulin 82%, and betazole 80%. Inhibition of food-stimulated gastric volume ranges from 30% to 65%. Pepsin and intrinsic factors are decreased, but serum gastrin is increased. Cimetidine does not change lower esophageal sphincter pressure, but it does block histamine-stimulated pressure increases.[19]

Adverse side effects (i.e., diarrhea, muscular pains, rashes, and dizziness) have been reported by 1% of patients given cimetidine for 8 weeks. These are usually mild and do not require stopping the drug use. Ileus has also been reported in burn patients who have received cimetidine.

Cimetidine therapy is indicated for short-term treatment of duodenal ulcer and pathologic hypersecretory conditions. Dosage and administration are as follows:
   1. Dosage:
      a. In children 20 to 40 mg/kg/day administered every 6 hours
      b. In adults 300 mg every 6 hours

2. Administration:
    a. Administered preferably by IV; may be diluted with 5% aqueous dextrose solution (D_5W) or Ionosol MB in D_5W; at least 20 ml of diluent infused over 15 to 30 minutes
    b. Cimetidine should be discontinued gradually

It has been shown in clinical studies that combined cimetidine and antacid therapy is more effective than either one alone in reducing gastric acidity. The addition of cimetidine reduces complications from antacids and the frequent interruption of gastric decompression. Concomitant antacid therapy is recommended for the 2 to 3 weeks that cimetidine is used for treatment.

The dosage for antacid therapy is as follows:

1. Aluminum hydroxide gel contains: Aluminum hydroxide, 320 mg/5 ml; sodium content, 6.9 mg/5 ml
2. Magnesium hydroxide-aluminum hydroxide contains: Aluminum hydroxide, 200 mg/5 ml; magnesium hydroxide, 200 mg/5 ml; simethicone, 20 mg/5 ml; sodium content, 3.9 mg/5 ml

Aluminum hydroxide may cause phosphate depletion, constipation, and with prolonged use, bone resorption, increased calcium absorption, and hypercalciuria.

Magnesium hydroxide often causes diarrhea. Toxicity may occur if a patient has renal failure. Magnesium hydroxide should not be used with patients who have nitrogen retention.

Surgical treatment. Any patient who has an unexplained fall in hematocrit, sudden increase in pulse, rapid elevation of blood urea nitrogen (BUN), bloody aspirate in the stomach from feeding tubes, or tarry or guaiac positive stools, should be considered for surgery to stop bleeding. Surgery may be required if conservative measures fail. If the patient has a stress ulcer requiring surgery, an operation should not be unduly delayed. Vagotomy and pyloroplasty or, preferably, vagotomy and hemigastrectomy should be performed. If the rate of bleeding can be ascertained to be the equivalent of one half the patient's blood volume within a 24-hour period, exploratory surgery should be performed.

Hypothermia

Incidence and cause. Hypothermia is normal in burn patients. Temperatures are generally 96° to 97° F (35.5° to 36° C) and can be even lower with exposure to a cold environment or extensive use of topical ice water. These external causes are aggravated by insensible water loss through the burn wound. This ranges between 0.5 to 3.5 ml with an average of 1.5 ml per percent of second- and third-degree burn per kilogram of body weight per 24 hours. For example, in a 70-kg patient with a 40% BSA burn, insensible water loss will be 4200 ml in 24 hours ($1.5 \times 70 \times 40$). The obligatory heat from evaporation can be calculated by multiplying this figure, 4200 ml, times 0.576 calories to give the caloric heat loss. This number, 2419, represents the heat lost from the patient with this extent and depth of burn. If the body does not increase its metabolic rate to compensate for this loss, body temperature cannot be maintained, and hypothermia will ensue.

Clinically, however, a combination of events occur. First, all of the wound is not equally exposed to the air and thus not entirely subject to these rates of insensible loss; i.e., bedding, dressing, and topical antimicrobial agents reduce this loss. Second, the metabolic rate increases to partially compensate for the deficit.

Diagnosis. The diagnosis of hypothermia can sometimes be confused with gram-negative sepsis, which is likely to cause hyperthermia. If possible, rectal temperatures are preferable to oral or axillary. Otherwise an esophageal monitor is indicated.

Treatment. Application of an occlusive dressing reduces the amount of insensible water loss. However, the dressing collects exudate and establishes a warm, rich media for the growth of bacteria, maceration of tissue, and the possible conversion from a second-degree burn to a full-thickness injury. External heat using a radiant heat source is recommended, but only to the degree that the patient is comfortable, usually in the low 90° F (32.2° C) range or at a point where health care personnel are slightly uncomfortable.

Catabolism

Catabolism occurs to a varying extent in all major burns. The causes include obligatory energy of evaporation, reaction to the burn injury, decreased nutrition, increased protein loss, and ileus. It is generally accepted that patients with major burns are best treated at first NPO, and that a degree of catabolism directly after the injury cannot be altered. However, some health care providers have proposed that enteric feeding through a nasoduodenal tube with a solution of 3.5% Aminosyn, 25% Polycose, and an appropriate addition of electrolytes and vitamins based on intravenous alimentation (IVH) solutions will achieve a positive nitrogen balance within 10 days. Patients should tolerate the enteric feedings well. A degree of hypermetabolism is also generally accepted as inevitable but an early nutritional program is mandatory.[15]

Hypermetabolism

The hypermetabolic response to burn injury is not significantly reduced when patients are comfortable, resting, or sleeping in a warm environment, and increased oxygen consumption cannot be explained by elevated body temperature. This does not support the contention that burn hypermetabolism is primarily the result of thermoregulatory drives. The increased heat production following injury is a consequence of an elevated metabolic state.

Insensible water loss

As discussed in Chapter 8, it is difficult to reduce the amount of insensible water loss with dressings without compromising control of burn wound sepsis. The pulmonary insensible loss can be somewhat reduced with the use of humidified air and proper ventilatory support, but not significantly.

Adrenal insufficiency

Demonstrable adrenal insufficiency rarely occurs in the burn patient, especially during the early postburn period. Because of the highly adverse side effects of adrenal steroid therapy, it should only be used with a specific laboratory diagnosis.

Normal cortisol ranges are: 7 to 20 μg/dl in the AM

3 to 15 μg/dl in the PM

Fever

Fever is not usually seen in the first few days postburn because invasive burn wound sepsis or pneumonitis needs more time to develop. Small febrile episodes are often masked by the enormous heat loss through the wound. Similar to other trauma states, atelectasis followed by urinary tract infection can occur early in the course, and all body fluid and its sources should be cultured before instituting therapy. In the burn patient it is especially important to carefully select specific antibiotics. It should also be noted that leukopenia is as frequent as leukocytosis with gram-negative infections, and therefore a negative or normal white blood cell count may not be as helpful as in other bacterial infections.[7,9,11]

Hemophilia

After early loading with cryoprecipitate, burned hemophiliacs do not require continued antihemophilic factor (AHF) because repair and restoration of vascular integrity in small vessels may occur as a result of platelet plugging and vessel retraction. Tissue thromboplastin may also contribute to clotting in burned hemophiliacs. AHF may be required if the patient needs an escharotomy in the early postburn period.[5]

Chemical intoxicants

When clinical and laboratory findings are not consistent with expected results, the likelihood of previously unrecognized chemical intoxication is strong. The most common causes are prescription or nonprescription medications, but it is not unusual to find that illegal drugs are the cause of clinical disparity. These are far ranging in their effects on the cardiopulmonary and nervous systems, and even their identification may not be helpful in managing the patient except to eliminate other causes. Treatment is close monitoring and specific pharmacologic response to clinical, but not necessarily laboratory, events.

Particularly in industrial fires, but increasingly in other conflagrations, chemical intoxication absorbed usually through the respiratory tract may be a factor. As discussed in Chapter 9, most of the clinical problems in these patients are related to nonspecific agents such as carbon monoxide, hypoxia, and irritating agents in general, but the treating physician should be aware of other possibilities and seek appropriate consultation.

Hepatitis, acquired immune deficiency syndrome, and disseminated intravascular coagulation

The transfusion risk of hepatitis (e.g., hepatitis A, hepatitis B, hepatitis non-A, hepatitis non-B, cytomegalovirus, Epstein-Barr virus) following transfusion is the same for burn patients receiving nonsterilized products (red blood cells, platelets, plasma, and cryoprecipitates) as for any other class of patients. Precise statistics about the number of patients who develop hepatitis following massive transfusions are not known. Approximately 5% to 10% of patients develop non-A or non-B hepatitis (most cases will be subclinical, but a significant number develop chronic liver disease and its sequelae); 0.6% have hepatitis (with another 1% converting blood serum without overt disease); and approximately 1% acquire cytomegalovirus. Hepatitis A and Epstein-Barr virus are rare causes of hepatitis following transfusion, and the latter is of no consequence when it does occur.

The risk of acquired immune deficiency syndrome (AIDS) following transfusion is currently extremely low. Data from the prescreening and pretesting era (late 1970s and early 1980s) suggest that the risk is approximately one case per 100,000 transfusions. Current data are incomplete and necessarily premature, but the National Institutes of Health suggest that one in 2.5 million transfusions transmit AIDS.

The best precaution to avoid developing disseminated intravascular coagulation is prevention of sepsis and hypovolemia. Treatment remains the treatment of the underlying cause. Heparinization and transfusion to replace consumed clotting factors are usually not necessary. When necessary, heparin doses should be given in amounts lower than those needed for thromboembolic disease.

SUMMARY

Each patient with a major thermal injury is a unique study. The medical practitioner has no set rules, only guidelines, based on broad knowledge of thermal injury pathophysiology coupled with a working understanding of all of the numerous medical and behavioral disciplines, particularly as they impact on developing effective treatment for the severely burned patient. At best, meeting the challenge of the thermally injured patient becomes an opportunity for a unique learning experience.

REFERENCES

1. Bingham, HG, et al: Burn diabetes: a review, J Burn Care 3:179, 1982.
2. Caffee, HH, and Bingham, HG: Leukopenia and silver sulfadiazine, J Trauma 22:586, 1982.
3. Deitch, EA, and Staats, RN: Child abuse through burning, J Burn Care 3:89, 1982.
4. Demling, RH, et al: Burn edema. II. Complications, prevention and treatment, J Burn Care 3:199, 1982.
5. Durtschi, MB, Counts, RB, and Heimbach, DM: The burned hemophiliac, J Trauma 20:706, 1980.
6. Durtschi, MB, et al: Burn injury in infants and young children, Surg Gynecol Obstet 150:651, 1980.
7. Halebian, P, et al: A burn center experience with toxic epidermal necrolysis, J Burn Care 4:176, 1983.
8. German, JC, Allyn, PA, and Barlett, RH: Pulmonary artery pressure monitoring in acute burn management, Arch Surg 106:788, 1973.
9. Gerow, FJ, and Weeder, RS: Medical aspects of the treatment of the burned patient, Med Clin North Am 48:1157, 1964.
10. Kempe, CH, and Helfer, RF: Helping the battered child and his family, Chicago, 1971, University of Chicago Press.
11. Kim, PS, et al: Stevens-Johnson syndrome and toxic epidermal necrolysis: a pathophysiologic review with recommendations for a treatment protocol, J Burn Care 4:91, 1982.
12. Lewis, PJ, and Zuker, RM: Childhood scald burns: an inquiry into severity, J Burn Care 3:95, 1982.
13. Libber, SM, and Stayton, DJ: Childhood burns reconsidered: the child, the family, and the burn injury, J Trauma 24:245, 1984.
14. Mancusi-Ungaro, HR, Jr, Tarbox, AR, and Wainwright, DJ: Post-traumatic stress disorder in electric burn patients, J Burn Care and Rehabil 7:521, 1986.
15. McArdle, AH, et al: Protection from catabolism in major burns: a new formula for the immediate enteral feeding of burn patients, J Burn Care 4:245, 1983.
16. Moran, KT, Kotowski, MP, and Munster, AM: Long-term disability following high-voltage electric hand injuries, J Burn Care and Rehabil 7:526, 1986.
17. Moritz, AR, and Henriques, FC, Jr: Studies of thermal injury. II. The relative importance of time and surface temperature in the causation of cutaneous burns, Am J Pathol 23:695, 1947.
18. Sasaki, TM, et al: The relationship of central venous and pulmonary artery catheter position to acute right-sided endocarditis in severe thermal injury, J Trauma 19:740, 1979.
19. Watson, WA, et al: Cimetidine in the prophylaxis of stress ulceration in severely burned patients, J Burn Care 4:260, 1983.

12 Special Types and Sites

OVERVIEW

Some types and sites of thermal injury require special attention. The clinician often renders the emergency care treatment required by having to deviate from, and many times abandon, the principles of resuscitation and wound care. Moreover, consultation and/or support in these special areas is in many instances by individuals who are both unfamiliar with the peculiarities of the thermal aspects of the injury and the problem(s) being targeted.

To provide a frame of reference for the treatment issues being addressed in special and unique areas, as well as to serve as exemplars for problems in areas not covered, the following causes and injury sites discussed in this chapter have been selected not only because they are examples of problems in areas not covered in this book, but also because they are important contributors to the mortality and morbidity rates relating to thermal injury.

SPECIAL CAUSES
Electrical injury[2,9,13,14]

Although electric shock produces a transtissue injury similar to that of the action of a microwave oven, its most dramatic effect is electrocution, which results in cardiac and respiratory arrest. However, flashburns from arcing, burns from the secondary ignition of clothing, major fractures from falls or myocardial infarctions caused by preexisting disease and/or stress, are more frequent and, fortunately, less damaging.

Although the first victim of industrial electrical injury was in 1879 in Lyon, France, and there was great fear in the 1880s when Thomas Edison first proposed wiring America's cities, the production of electricity over the last 100 years has resulted in only a relatively small increase in deaths that can be directly or indirectly related to electrical injury.

Incidence. The most frequent electrically caused thermal injuries that do occur fall into three general categories: occupational, children, and adults.

Occupational. Most occupational injuries occur in males in the prime working age group. Not unexpectedly, many of these are employed by the electric companies or represent untrained, poorly supervised or careless construction workers.

Children. Examples of categories into which children with thermal injuries fall are: (1) infants who frequently bite on electrical cords or place their fingers in electrical sockets, (2) youngsters playing near power lines, or (3) children who are injured by faulty or improperly designed toys. Such toy injuries, although unusual, should be promptly reported to the Consumer Product Safety Commission (CPSC), Washington, DC, or to their local office.

Fig. 12-1 shows a third-degree electrical burn of the corner of the mouth in a child who has bitten on an electrical wire. Note the depth of the burn, which extends through the deep muscle or oris orbicularis. Although this is a common injury in children, reconstruction can be difficult; treatment, usually by a plastic surgeon, requires early full debridement and reconstruction. Late treatment usually results in severe functional and cosmetic deformities.

Adults. Adult injuries occur almost exclusively in males. They occur frequently in individuals working on "do it yourself" projects, often involving TV antennas. Each year there are several reported electric blanket, electric heating pad, and electric hairdryer or appliance burns reported. But compared to their vast use, the number of injuries is almost insignificant, and the burns are of the minor cutaneous type rather than the unique electrical transtissue injury.

Characteristics. It is important to understand how electrical burns differ from other burn injuries.

Amperage is the term used for the rate of flow of electrons. Every time 6242×10^{15} electrons pass a given point in one second, 1 A of current has passed. It is the current that can kill or hurt the victim. One ampere is roughly equivalent to the amount of current flowing through a 100-watt light bulb.

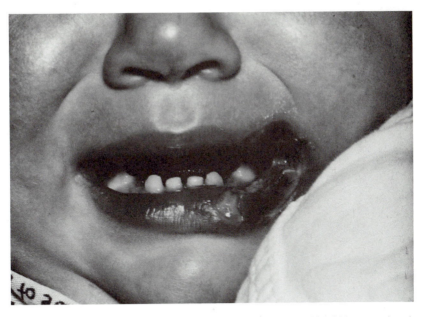

Fig. 12-1. Third-degree burn of corner of mouth in child caused by biting an electric cord.

An electrical potential or voltage of 10 V or less is considered low-tension voltage, whereas a voltage of more than 10 V is high-tension voltage.

High-tension wires usually carry alternating current. Alternating current is more dangerous than direct current—the alternating causes tetanic spasms, which make the victim grip the electrodes more firmly, increasing the insult and the danger to the heart and respiratory centers.

The skin resistance is encountered primarily in the stratum corneum, which serves as an insulator for the body. The voltage gradient in skin cannot be increased indefinitely and breaks down at low voltages.

Exposure of the skin to 50 V for 6 or 7 seconds results in blisters that have a considerably diminished electrical resistance. The resistance offered by the dermis is low, as is that of almost all internal tissues except bone, which is a poor conductor of electricity. In most electrical injuries the voltage remains constant and the effect depends upon the amperage, type of current, resistance at the point of contact, the path through the body, the duration of the contact, and individual susceptibility.

Humans are extremely sensitive to very small electric currents because of their highly developed nervous systems. Body resistance varies. The callous palm may reach 1,000,000 Ω; but the average skin resistance is 5000 Ω, and in most skin it is as small as 1000 Ω.

Mechanism. How a true electrical burn causes injury has not been fully defined, but it does result in fibrillation of the heart, brain injury, and coagulation of the blood vessels and other tissues.

Electrothermal burns are a result of the heat generated, and the temperature may approximate 2500° C. It is generally believed that under ordinary conditions arcing occurs in a high-tension line approximately 1 inch for every 20,000 V; but once the arc is established, it can exist or be drawn out over longer distances.

The degree of tissue damage in an electrical injury is proportional to the intensity of current that passes through the victim: As stated in Ohm's law (below), the resistance of tissues varies to the flow of current. In order of decreasing magnitude, current passes through bone, fat, tendon, skin, muscle, blood, and nerve.

If

$$I \text{ (current)} = \frac{E \text{ (voltage)}}{R \text{ (resistance)}}$$

since

$$P \text{ (power)} = E \times I$$

then

$$P = \frac{E}{R} = I R$$

The thermal component of an electrical injury does not vary linearly with the voltage, but as the square of the applied voltage or as the square of the current flow. For example, doubling the voltage (for a given resistance) quadruples the power absorbed by the resistance (victim), and power, not current, per se, is a more accurate indicator of heat generated.

Hence, a 2400-V power line will feed 400 times more power (heat) into a resistance than a 120-V power line.

Flame burns result from the ignition of clothing. Depending on the type of clothing, these secondary burns can be considerable.

Special consideration must be given to the severe injury to the heart and respiratory centers and to the fact that the injury is deep, often involving bone, muscle, and other structures. Deep injury is often more serious than that which occurs to the skin at the point of entrance and exit. In addition, other injuries frequently are related to the severe convulsions, i.e., dislocations, fractures.

There are four factors that differentiate electrical burns from usual thermal injuries: direct effect on the myocardium; direct effect on the brain stem; deep destruction due to intense heat; and thrombus formation.

Treatment. In a study by Parshley and associates,[2] flame and arc burns are classified as noncurrent injuries, and current burns as current injuries. Current injury results when a high current passes through the body from a contact point to one or more places where it reaches an area of lower potential or ground. Entrance and exit sites are usually identifiable at various distances apart on the body surface. They can be quite small and remote from each other and victims must be carefully examined to determine "in or out" for this type of injury. Exit site findings also give some indication of the pathway and extent of an insidiously deep injury that must be treated.

The first aid for electrical trauma, listed in order of priority, is as follows:

1. Prevent further injury
2. CPR
3. Stop hemorrhage
4. Splint fractures
5. Treat burns
6. Transport

There are three major differences between care of the electric burn and other thermal injuries:

1. The need to prevent further electrical injury, not only to the victim but more often to the rescuers
2. The immediate need for CPR
3. An appreciation for the deep tissue injury, often without extensive cutaneous involvement

Both noncurrent and current injuries can occur in the same patient. An aggressive approach is to decompress muscle compartments and debride necrotic tissue; occasional amputation may be necessary. Aggressive treatment may prevent some of the devastating disabilities and systemic illnesses characteristic of these injuries such as renal failure. Autogenous grafts should rarely be used initially, because most need to be reexplored and further debrided within several days.

Lightning

Incidence. It is estimated that in the United States, between 110 and 600 lightning deaths occur each year. The exact figure has been difficult to establish, but it is clear that more direct deaths occur from lightning than from any other weather phenomenon. Despite this incidence, two thirds of those involved in lightning strikes make a complete recovery, probably because most of the survivors are not actually struck by lightning, but receive an electric shock by being in the vicinity.[1,11,15,16]

Effect. Many organ systems can be involved in an electrical injury. Cardiac arrhythmias are commonly seen following injury; ST-segment elevation, T-wave inversion, and atrial and ventricular arrhythmias occur during the acute phase; and transient hypertension has been reported.

Gastrointestinal complications are not unique, but are similar to those found with major trauma or burns. Although second-, third-, and fourth-degree burns may occur, most are superficial.

Treatment. Lightning burns tend to be skin-deep only and should be treated as any other burn wound. Rarely do they bear any similarity to the deep electrical injuries previously described. Treat cardiac injury and hypertension as required; use cardiopulmonary resuscitation if necessary.

Chemical burns

Unless chemicals generate or are associated with heat production, they do not cause burns that are similar in effect to those of thermal injury. The injury is limited to the area of contact, unless absorption of the chemical has taken place. This occurrence is rare, and unlike thermal burns, chemical burns do not cause systemic pathophysiologic changes. Much of this may be due to the usually limited body surface area involved, and in this respect treatment is more closely akin to that of the minor burn in which function and cosmesis are of primary concern.

Common types of injury. These types of injuries generally fall into two types: occupational, including those associated with laboratory and cleaning work; and those accidentally occurring in the home. In the latter case the injury is usually minor, whereas in the former the injury may be profound or even fatal.

Diagnosis. Although the diagnosis of chemical burns is usually obvious, the cause and the extent can be obscure. The alkali burns are notorious for their persistent action caused by their release and reattachment to the protein in the tissue. Acid burns can also be insidious, often continuing to damage the skin while hidden by clothing.

Treatment. The first specific treatment following rescue and extrication is the rapid application of copious amounts of water. Although desirable, the use of neutralizing solutions and even the removal of clothing should not delay in any way the use of water. In the case of alkaline chemical injury, water will not suffice and will need to be rapidly supplanted by an acid solution, but in the early stages water is usually far more available.

With some chemicals, notably those containing phosphorous, water is strictly contraindicated. These chemicals are rarely found outside the military or clearly marked areas in industry. Some awareness is prudent. To enhance this prudence, the Chemical Manufacturers' Association (Washington, D.C. 20037) has established a Community Awareness and Emergency Response (CAER) program.

Following the application of water to neutralize and dilute the chemicals, the clothing should be gently removed. Often parenteral analgesics will be required before this is possible. The wound should be examined, cleansed with an iodophor or hexachlorophene solution, and treated with topical silver sulfadiazine or Sulfa-mylon.

No systemic antibiotics are indicated unless identifiable infection is already present. Tetanus immunization procedures should be performed. Somewhat similar to a thermal burn, it is often exceedingly difficult to determine the depth of the injury until 24 to 48 hours have elapsed. Therefore no definitive debridement should be planned at least until that time.

Only if necessary to protect the wound from further injury or for splinting should a dressing—plain gauze only—be applied.

Care following injury is again similar to that for the minor burn, i.e., analgesics, twice daily washes, and redressing and/or application of a topical agent. All patients should be reexamined at least in 24 hours.

Radiation burns and reactions

Radiation burns have been best described most recently as radiation reactions. Similar to thermal injuries, they do interfere with the functions of the skin. But unlike them, they do not permit increased insensible water loss and bacterial invasion, nor markedly increased absorption of medication or similar systemic changes except as related to the radiation.

In the United States the incidence of radiation skin reaction has decreased with the use of improved sources and better methodology. There is seldom a need for emergency treatment and the reaction, like the primary disease, is a chronic issue.

In treating radiation reactions of the skin, a number of principles are related not only to care of the thermally burned patient, but to wound care in general. Most notable is the need for frequent cleansing and the application of topical antimicrobials, preferably in a nonpetrolatum base. In the event of wound sepsis, principles of debridement and delayed closure are also applicable.

SPECIAL AREAS
Eye[3,4,17]

Types of injuries. In a recent study corneal ulceration was reported as the most common ocular problem, occurring in 86% of the patients with an eye injury. Corneal perforation occurred in 14% of the injuries and was by far the most serious injury. Since corneal perforations are often related to other extensive injuries, 50% of the patients with perforation died. The most prevalent infecting organism in these cases was coagulase positive *Staphylococcus aureus*. Previous ophthalmologic concentration has been focused primarily on the recognition and treatment of ectropion and of corrosive injury.

Diagnosis. The diagnosis must be made early before edema makes examination exceedingly difficult. Rapid assessment to ascertain the intactness of the globe and to observe the glistening polish of the cornea and the position, shape, and size of the pupil should be followed by an ophthalmoscopic examination.

A gross evaluation of visual acuity immediately on admission can later prove to be invaluable. For similar reasons, if there is any indication of damage to the eye, including eyelids, examination by an ophthalmologist within the first several hours is highly desirable.

Immediate treatment. The immediate treatment of burns of the eyelid is essentially the same as that for burns that occur in other areas. The periorbital areas should be gently cleansed with saline-saturated gauze pads to remove the loose debris, necrotic material, coagulum, and/or foreign material. Topical steroidal eye ointments may be used to keep the lids soft and pliable along with topical anti-microbial agents.

If the initial examination indicates a mushy, soft globe or penetrating wound, a protective "shield" should be devised and placed over the eye.

Coagulated epithelium and corneal burns are recognized by the loss of the usual perfect transparency of that structure. Epithelial defects can be readily seen by applying some fluorescein stain to the cornea. A defect in the epithelium is indeed a "mini ulcer" and requires vigorous treatment in terms of prevention of desiccation and infection.

A misshapen pupil is usually the sign of a perforated or ruptured globe. A constricted but round pupil is indicative of iritis. There is some traumatic iritis in all burns. This produces photophobia and can be treated with topical steroid and cycloplegic drops.

If the eyelids alone are burned, a standard eye pressure dressing may be applied. For generalized burns no viable skin would be available for attachment of the dressing. Sometimes a headroll-type dressing may be used.

None of the perforated corneas reported responded to ophthalmic treatment. Initial closure of perforations is more successful with conjunctival flaps.

For the treatment of infection, surface microbial cultures and appropriate anti-microbials, soft contact lenses, and patching are effective when used in conjunction with moisturizing barrier agents. Cycloplegic agents offer symptomatic relief of pain in some cases.

Although tarsorrhaphies have been recommended for protection of the cornea in patients with eyelid burns, they are not required and can lead to irreparable damage to the eyelids. During the early edema phase, the eyelids are swollen shut; thus the cornea is protected. Once the eyelid has healed or been grafted, the subsequent contracture can lead to ectropion and exposure of the cornea. In these cases tarsorrhaphy has not proven effective. Exposure keratitis, chronic conjunctivitis, and infection are serious and unusual complications. They can best be prevented by early eyelid reconstruction.

A deep second-degree burn of the face involving the eyelid is shown in Fig. 12-2 4 days following injury. Note the severe edema that can persist for several weeks, making eye care exceedingly difficult.

Indications for consultation. Corneal infections caused by *Pseudomonas* are not uncommon and can be disastrous. Early recognition and consultation are mandatory. Similarly, any indication of uveitis or acute glaucoma should be diagnosed early by frequent examination for conjunctival injection, changes in the pupil, and deterioration of visual acuity. To ensure the detection of these events early, the eyes must be fully examined, including a vision test and ophthalmoscopic examination.

Instructions to patient. The patient should be informed about the essential nature of the polishing and protecting action of the eyelids. Contracture of the eyelids

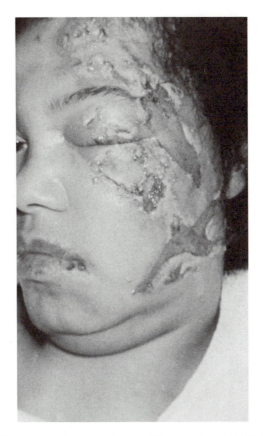

Fig. 12-2. Deep second-degree burns of face and eyelids 4 days postburn.

results in the loss of both these functions. This leads to desiccation, followed by ulceration, which in turn is followed by perforation. The eye itself must be kept moist and protected around the clock. Numerous drops and ointments are available. Protective devices can be fashioned in order to provide a moist chamber over the eye. Topical eye anesthetics slow down epithelization of the cornea and thus should not be used routinely. Pain should be controlled by systemic medications. Reassurance of both the family and patient is particularly important in the early phase when the eyelids are often completely closed.

Face and ears

The face and ears represent a unique challenge. Because of its abundant blood supply, the facial area is particularly resistant to infection and apt to heal readily by

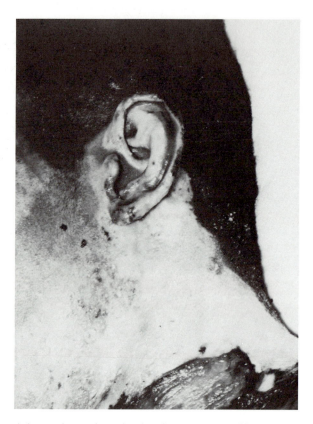

Fig. 12-3. Second-degree burn of ear that has been converted by pressure necrosis to third-degree injury involving cartilage.

epithelialization. However, deep burns of these regions are often ominous signs of a severe inhalation or otherwise extensive injury. Therefore treatment because of other serious and concomitant injuries is usually conservative management of the wounds. Early full-thickness debridement and even tangential excision are generally not recommended. Open treatment, frequent washings, and topical antimicrobials are the treatment modes of choice. The results are usually rather surprisingly good.

One exception is the ears: there is no subcutaneous tissue on the ears, and the underlying cartilage is easily involved in both the burn injury or in any subsequent invasive sepsis. Particular care should be taken to prevent pressure necrosis. Although the frequency of this occurrence can be reduced by the use of soft, padded dressings, the increased likelihood of sepsis under this condition requires extra caution in local wound care. Fig. 12-3 shows a second-degree burn of the ear 7 days after injury. Note the involvement and deformity of the cartilage secondary to pressure necrosis.

Hand

Evaluation of wound depth. Estimation of the burn depth is critical. It is well accepted that, if the burn is first degree or superficial second degree (i.e., a wound that will heal completely within 3 weeks), treatment should be nonsurgical.[5-8,10]

If the burn appears deeper (i.e., deep second-degree or third-degree), as soon as possible following resuscitation, generally within 3 days, it should be excised tangentially with grafting to reach viable bleeding tissue. The wounds should be covered immediately with split-thickness skin. Because of the open gaps, mesh grafts should not be used, if at all possible.

The difficult treatment decision occurs when there are mainly superficial second-degree burns with a few small areas of deeper injury. In these cases early excision and grafting, even with the apparent sacrifice of a small amount of skin that might heal, will often give a better functional result. The other problem arises when the patient has a massive cutaneous total BSA burn, often with concomitant inhalation injury and hand burns, and in whom a surgical procedure during the first few days would be hazardous. In this instance it is best to follow the general principle that a patient should be stable before surgery should be performed, unless the patient is in imminent danger of deteriorating and the surgery planned might be a stabilizing factor. With regard to hand burns, it is important to remember that saving the hands is not as important as saving the life.

On the other hand, the all-too-frequent occurrence to "procrastinate" (i.e., defer surgery) until the patient is "better" and has an excellent lifesaving prognosis frequently results in increased sepsis or at least in inflammation around the joint capsules, the tendons and tendon sheaths, and a markedly poor function capability.

Local care. As soon as the patient is better, early debridement and grafting are beneficial; however, it is doubtful whether enzymatic debridement is of much value. Local care consists of washing the wound thoroughly under sterile precautions and using a mild antiseptic solution, debriding obviously necrotic tissue and applying either silver nitrate solution, Sulfamylon or silver sulfadiazine.

Although open care is generally preferable with the latter two treatments, it is usually necessary to dress the hand wound to encourage functioning. The dressing should be changed at least twice daily, the hand bathed, and active and passive motion started as soon as possible, usually within a few days.

Dressing and splinting. There is a continuing debate surrounding the adverse effects of dressing and splinting—which in itself acts as a dressing—and the need to splint in order to prevent contractures. An alternative is the use of wire rods and dynamic action traction. This method, however, has not been widely accepted. The most common procedure is simple splinting in position of function, although splinting in this position in a burn injury is also open to debate, since the contractures that occur are usually those of hyperextension of the first metacarpal phalangeal joint with flexion of the phalangeal joints. A more functional splint would seem to be one of full extension. In either instance, it is most important to start frequent active and passive motion as soon as the edema permits. The splints should also be removed at least twice daily to permit examination and care of the burn wound.

Grafting. Early tangential excision and immediate autografting is an excellent method of treating deep second-degree burns of the hands. However, only after careful evaluation should patients with large, life-threatening thermal injuries be selected for this procedure. The use of mesh grafts at this point leaves open areas requiring more careful wound care, but the mesh graft does provide more flexibility.

Full-thickness dorsal hand and digit burns still result in serious acute and chronic functional disability, although early surgical excision, grafting, and aggressive physical and occupational therapy have minimized and/or decreased some of the expected dysfunctional sequelae.

In a study by Goodwin and associates,[7] a prospective evaluation was conducted by 164 burned hands of patients consecutively admitted (mean age 29); the mean burn size was 37% BSA. Early surgery was shown to produce no adverse effect on survival. Excision and grafting of hands with deep dermal burns, whether early or late, offered no advantage in maintaining hand function over physical therapy and primary healing. Likewise, hands with more superficial burns responded equally to surgical and nonsurgical treatment.

Although early excision and grafting of hands with third-degree burns tended to produce poorer results than did initial nonsurgical care and late grafting, the differences are just outside the range of significance. Early excision and grafting of selected third-degree injuries of the hands may be indicated in patients with small total BSA burns to shorten hospital stay. However, early surgical intervention in patients with massive burns should be directed toward area coverage, not necessarily toward coverage of the hand.

Perineum

Burns of the perineum are not uncommon in either the very young or the very old. Hot water scalds are the most common cause. In children, they occur most frequently from inadvertently sitting in a tub that is too hot or from child abuse.

In the elderly the burns can also occur with the same rapidity as with children if the elderly person sits in a tub of hot water and is unable to move fast enough to prevent a major burn. The hot water temperature in elderly housing is controlled by federal regulation to no more than 125° F (51.6° C), but even at this temperature, the elderly or children may be burned before they can extricate themselves.

Burns of the perineum are also seen in patients with a flame burn, but in these cases they are usually associated with severe and extensive deep cutaneous injury.

Special dangers. The special dangers are primarily concerned with sepsis, either because of self-contamination or because of the difficulty in treating patients with burns of the perineum. These patients should be admitted because care is difficult at home and close observation is important during the early postburn period.

Sepsis can readily cause conversion to third-degree or full-thickness burns by destroying viable cells in the dermis or dermal structures that might otherwise not be recognized as being still viable.

Use of catheters. Unless the patient is fully continent and there is no burn of the genitalia, it is most important to use an indwelling catheter during the initial 48 to 96 hours. In children, this may not be necessary, and there is often some hesitancy because of the frequent occurrence of urinary sepsis and/or urethral strictures. In these cases it is best to leave the infant exposed rather than to risk chaffing by a diaper, which will cause further injury and lead to maceration of the tissue, sepsis, and delayed wound healing or conversion to third-degree burns.

Prevention of sepsis. Sepsis is the major problem associated with burns of the perineum. Continually contaminated, moist with a rich media of exudate, and pressured between the weight of the body and sterile sheet covering a plasticized mattress, the burned perineum presents the ideal opportunity for a rapid growth of bacteria. Prevention of sepsis has to be directed toward the following factors:

1. It must be recognized that, short of establishing a colostomy, which used to be routine but is no longer used as frequently, there is no way to prevent repeated contamination. Therefore special attention must be directed toward the other factors that promote bacterial growth and invasive sepsis. This can be done by reducing the number of bacteria in the contaminant by frequent washing and application of one of the topical antimicrobial agents such as Sulfamylon or silver sulfadiazine; and by frequent removal, by bathing and washing, of the accumulated exudate and reducing the maceration by exposure and ambulation or frequent turning.
2. There should be recognition that sepsis to some degree is inevitable, and early attention should be paid toward coverage.

Treatment. The treatment is focused on prevention of sepsis and early coverage as described above. Dressing of any type is not practical.

It should also be recognized that the sheet, and the standard plasticized mattress on which the patient is lying is de facto functioning as a dressing and one without a layer for the absorption of fluids that readily collect and contribute to the maceration and subsequent sepsis. If possible, the patient should be kept off the burn site or at least frequently rotated.

Washing several times a day, preferably in a tub bath, is highly recommended. Since the wound cannot be kept either isolated or free of exudate, every effort should be directed toward reducing both the number of bacteria in the contamination and the media in which they grow.

Intentional obstipation or an antibiotic bowel preparation is not recommended, but copious diarrheal stools must be avoided. This can best be accomplished by a low-residue diet and administration of stool softeners.

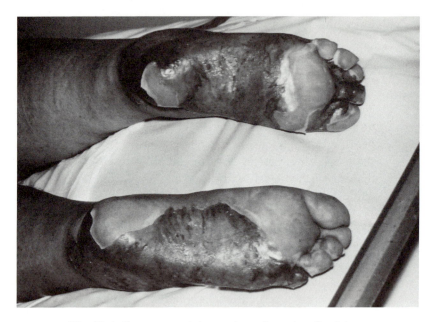

Fig. 12-4. Deep second-degree burn 5 weeks after injury.

Feet[18]

Burns of the feet can occur from hot water, by contact, or by flame. If they are caused by flame, they portend a particularly severe thermal injury, since the soles of the feet are not burned except under dire circumstances. Occasionally, severe burns of the sole of the feet are seen following stepping on a hot object such as stones previously used for a clambake.

Although the sole of the foot is thick and more resistant than other types of skin to thermal injury, it does not graft well. If full thickness is involved that will require pedicle flaps, these are also not satisfactory. Nevertheless, it is most important to prevent sepsis and conversion to third degree.

An example of a deep second-degree burn of the soles of the feet is shown in Fig. 12-4. This burn, which was treated conservatively for 5 weeks, demonstrates the gradual sloughing of the thick, burned epidermis and reveals "well healed" epithelium.

The use of early tangential excision and grafting is often very helpful, but the very circumstances that caused the burn, particularly if it involves other areas of the body, will frequently preclude an early surgical procedure or even the use of available skin for other than lifesaving maximum coverage. However, in prioritizing areas to be covered, a patient unable to stand for a long period of time can rapidly develop, or exacerbate, complications that could be fatal.

REFERENCES

1. Apfelberg, DB, Masters, FW, and Robinson, DW: Pathophysiology and treatment of lightning injuries, J Trauma 14:453, 1974.
2. Baxter, CR: Present concepts in the management of major electrical injury, Surg Clin North Am 50:1401, 1970.
3. Burns, CL, and Chylack, LT, Jr: Thermal burns: the management of thermal burns of the lids and globes, Ann Ophthalmol 11:1358, 1979.
4. Frank, DH, Wachtel, T, and Frank, HA: The early treatment and reconstruction of eyelid burns, J Trauma 23:874, 1983.
5. Frist, W, et al: Long-term functional results of selective treatment of hand burns, Am J Surg 149:516, 1985.
6. Gant, TD: The early enzymatic debridement and grafting of deep dermal burns to the hand, Plast Reconstr Surg 66:185, 1980.
7. Goodwin, CW, et al: Prospective study of burn wound excision of the hands, J Trauma 23:510, 1983.
8. Hunt, JL, and Sato, RM: Early excision of full-thickness hand and digit burns: factors affecting morbidity, J Trauma 22:414, 1982.
9. Layton, TB, et al: Multiple spinal fractures from electrical injury, J Burn Care 5:373, 1984.
10. Levine, BA, et al: Efficacy of tangential excision and immediate autografting of deep second-degree burns of the hand, J Trauma 19:670, 1979.
11. McCrady-Kahn, VL, and Kahn, AM: Lightning burns, J Burn Care 3:59, 1982.
12. Merrel, SW, et al: Full-thickness skin grafting for contact burns of the palm in children, J Burn Care Rehabil 7:501, 1986.
13. Nichter, LS, et al: Injuries due to commercial electric current, J Burn Care 5:124, 1984.
14. Parshley, PF, et al: Aggressive approach to the extremity damaged by electric current, Am J Surg 150:78, 1985.
15. Scheulen, JJ, and Munster, AM: The lightning injury, J Burn Care 4:101, 1983.
16. Strasser, EJ, Davis, RM, and Menchey, MJ: Lightning injuries, J Trauma 17:315, 1977.
17. Walters, MJ, and Lowell, GG: Corneal problems in burned patients, J Burn Care 3:367, 1982.
18. Zuker, RM, et al: Effective management of deep scald burns to the feet, J Burn Care 5:288, 1984.

13 Disaster Burn Care

OVERVIEW

Major developments in the treatment of the burn patient, even if applied with limited resources, will result in a mortality rate closely approaching the generally accepted level for a nondisaster situation. The knowledge that this improved care is available for the thermally injured patient in a disaster should do much to dispel the perpetual pessimism associated with this topic.[1,5,7,10,12,14,15] This chapter is primarily directed toward the resuscitation phase and the pregrafting care of the burn wound in a mass casualty situation.

MEDICAL DISASTER DEFINITION

Probably no other injury concerns disaster planners more than thermal injury, yet very little is written that is of help in either the planning or the actual delivery of care in a catastrophic situation. In such a situation, particularly when there is a substantial discrepancy between the need and the medical resources to meet that need, austere medical care is required if mortality and morbidity are to be minimized.

Of immediate concern is the ability to predict the scale of involvement, particularly the likelihood of large numbers of burn patients. In this regard, most disaster situations can be divided into several categories: natural disasters such as earthquakes, hurricanes, and volcanic eruptions; armed conflict such as large-scale nuclear and large- or small-scale conventional warfare; terrorist activities; and industrial accidents. Specific instances such as airplane accidents and terrorist activities can overlap several of these categories.

In general, only armed conflict involving large-scale armored warfare or bombings with napalm or other incendiaries and the fires that are caused by these conflicts result in large numbers of burn casualties. The conventional small-scale conflict, as well as various terrorist activities, do not usually result in many burn injuries. Similarly, natural disasters cause only minimal injuries or death, and rarely are there many burn victims.

In contrast, survivors of small plane accidents are often severely burned and have smoke inhalation injury. Although survivors of large plane crashes also have burns and smoke inhalation injury that complicate their other injuries, the outcome, like that in natural disasters, is usually survival without serious injury or death.

It is probably easiest to determine the number of thermal injury victims in an industrial accident. In addition, these cases are very often complicated by a smoke inhalation injury, frequently of the nonsmoke chemical inhalation type.

On the basis of the large-scale conventional warfare analysis of World Wars I and II, it has been accepted for planning purposes that in any disaster victims will be distributed in the four basic triage categories as follows: 20% immediate, 20% delayed, 20% expectant, and 40% minimal. However, this injury ratio seldom exists; nevertheless, other factors that affect the ability to provide care will necessitate the implementation of an operational plan at varying levels of austerity.

AUSTERE MEDICAL CARE
Frame of reference

The effective implementation of an austere medical care system requires a command structure that can deploy health care resources in the rigorous manner needed for handling a mass casualty situation. For its most effective implementation, it is essential not to create a new system, including terminology, but to join with the health care delivery systems in the public and private domains, as well as those in the armed forces, the public health services, the Federal Emergency Assistance Agency (FEMA), and the recently formed National Disaster Medical System (NDMS).[3,10,11,14]

Austerity levels

Sutherland[13] in 1981 and Orr[9] in 1983 described a systems analysis to delineate different combat situations according to the predictability of the outcome. This system provides a frame of reference for implementing austere medical care levels for disaster situations. The levels are: determinate or austerity level I; moderately stochastic or austerity level II; severely stochastic or austerity level II; and indeterminate or austerity level IV.

In a determinate situation (level I) the outcome is generally predictable, and the level of austerity to be practiced is minimal and temporary; whereas in a moderately stochastic or austerity level II mode there are temporary unknowns and shortages that imply that a more austere level of medical care must be adhered to.

In the severely stochastic situation (austerity level III), unknowns and/or severe limitations of resources exist to a level that there is major doubt as to the outcome.

In the event of an indeterminate or level IV occurrence, no predictable outcome or readily foreseeable solutions exist; thus only the most austere care can be given. When it becomes known that either resupply or patient evacuation will occur shortly, the level of care can be increased.

Triage of burn victims

The thermally injured patients are grouped into the same four categories according to treatment required as all other patients in a disaster situation, whether they are injured or suffering an illness: immediate, delayed, expectant, and minimal.

1. The immediate care category encompasses those patients who require immediate care or they will die. It can also include those who require immediate care to prevent deterioration to a moribund state.
2. The delayed category refers to those who require major care, but are stable and not in immediate danger of dying or deteriorating.
3. In the expectant category are those patients who, under the prevailing circumstances, are not expected to live. They do receive care, but only what is absolutely necessary for maintaining the maximum humane treatment relative to the available resources.
4. The patients who receive minimal care have minimal injury or illness and are in no danger of dying, but they may be at some functional or cosmetic risk.

Use of trauma scores

The application of trauma or injury severity scores may be useful, but only if the guidelines and scoring procedures can be readily understood and implemented. In this format burn thermal injury patients are classified with all other victims, both injured and ill. At the present time, specific care levels pertaining to burn victims have not been determined with the degree of certainty required for ensuring a minimal acceptable level of validity. It appears reasonable to assume that, once an adequate data base has been established, burn trauma scores will be of value in disaster burn management.[2,4]

FACTORS AFFECTING AUSTERITY OF CARE

Many factors affect the level of austere care that can be practiced. These factors vary in importance with both the overall situation and their relation to each other. A clear understanding and working knowledge of them is essential for effective decision making. Accordingly, an overview of primary factors to be considered in a mass casualty situation requiring austere medical care is presented in the following paragraphs.

Numbers of patients

Knowing the number of patients to be expected, and when, is essential. However, a reliable estimate of the number of casualties is usually not available during the very early stages of a disaster. Nevertheless, continual approximations of the number of patients to be expected is imperative, since these numbers are the basis for updating the level of care that can be prudently rendered.

Severity of injuries

This factor is the most variable, depending on the cause of the disaster. Estimations from the field are often wildly exaggerated because of the visual aspects of a burn injury, the drama of the situation, and the absence of a plan. Although any information from the field is helpful and should be actively sought, the severity of the injuries is most often determined at the medical facility triage site.

Types of injuries

The burn patients in a disaster often have a number of different types of injuries or diseases that affect both the level and type of care. Although the cutaneous burn may be the most dramatic, it may not be the most critical matter requiring attention.

Thermal. The type of thermal burn (e.g., scald, flame, electrical, or contact) often indicates the depth and extent of the burn and thus the amount of shock or other possible complications involved.

Smoke inhalation. The presence of even a limited smoke inhalation injury, when combined with a cutaneous burn, cardiopulmonary disease, or industrial toxic inhalation injury, can alter the prognosis.

Chemical. The presence of chemical burns and the toxicity caused by chemicals in an industrial accident can affect both the rescue attempts and the care that can be given.

Radiologic. Similar to chemical contamination, radiation injuries can rapidly overwhelm the capacity of a facility to provide any level of care. Planning for simple decontamination procedures such as water washing and isolation of contaminated clothing and supplies is essential. Personnel must be aware of the possibility of radiation hazards, particularly in the civilian sector; radioactive substances are usually present in many laboratories, hospitals, and in a variety of industries where least suspected.

Presence of other injuries or diseases. The presence of other major injuries, particularly those resulting in alterations of cardiopulmonary function or hypovolemic shock, can greatly affect the prognosis of the thermally injured patient. Similarly, diseases such as those of the cardiopulmonary and genitourinary systems adversely affect outcome. Thus the cutaneous burn injury can become secondary, and patients must be triaged and treated on the basis of their primary dysfunctions.

Extended care

Although an in-depth discussion of extended care does not fall within the scope of this chapter, resources may have to be considered for an extended and undetermined period. Obviously, knowledge of the duration that care must be given and the time or distance involved, including the resources available for transport for providing further care, are key inputs to determining the level of austerity to practice.

Medical personnel

Allocation. The most critical item in an austere medical practice situation is immediate access to and use of experienced medical personnel. They should be clearly identified and accorded key roles in handling triage. Many trained and experienced medical care personnel, including those involved in emergency room care, are not experienced with the provision of austere care. This lack of experience is evident by the triaging of too many patients into the immediate category and thus "wasting" high-priority medical supplies that are urgently required elsewhere.

Stress management. The care, feeding, and rest of medical personnel are often neglected. Organization into teams, sharing of responsibility, and enforced rest periods are mandatory if continued care is to be given to the patients. Like other resources, there must be a plan for rationing, and it must be enforced by a command structure that has been established preferably before the crisis occurs.

Although the physical well-being is a primary consideration, it has been demonstrated that in catastrophic situations an intense emotional reaction has the potential to interfere with the ability of medical personnel to function, either at the scene or later. An example of this stress phenomenon has been described by Honig[6] in an analysis of the 1986 Cerritos air disaster. Koenigsburg[8] has presented stress to be a critical factor in reducing the overall effectiveness of rescue efforts in the Agency for International Development's rescue programs.

Selection. Ideally, personnel positions and their qualifications should be identified before the onset of a catastrophe. Since the ideal is rarely evidenced, personnel identification and selection should at the very least be performed immediately when the alert of an impending disaster is received. It is necessary to start with the identification of experienced team leaders and organize the disaster effort by assignment of the most experienced to perform the triage followed by assignment of the next most experienced to the immediate care and those least experienced to the delayed care areas. Everyone with experience must be both a teacher and treatment administrator at all available opportunities, including "idle periods."

There is also a need to identify those personnel who can fill the essential support roles such as security, maintenance, transport, and communication.

Number. The actual number of medical personnel available, regardless of their training in mass casualty care, will have a major impact on the care to be given in a disaster situation. Subject to proper use, augmentation with nonmedical personnel can greatly expand the capability of austere medical efforts. However, the traditional physician manpower available can be augmented by co-related medical care professions such as dentists, veterinarians, and optometrists, many of whom have received mass casualty care training in the military service or in the 1960s through the Department of Defense Medical Education for National Defense (MEND) program.[4a,5a,6a]

Regardless of the number and type of personnel involved, written, preprinted protocols for each personnel level and type of care are invaluable.

Facilities

The type, location, and number of facilities are major contributing factors in determining the austerity level of care that must be practiced. Facilities can vary from a hospital to alternative fixed facilities such as a school building, tents, or even the open field. Shelter from the elements is important to survival, as is access to sanitation. Personnel with experience in this area—particularly those at the technical level such as plumbers, carpenters, and general mechanics—are often in short supply in a medical facility and should be quickly identified and included at all levels of planning and operation for implementing an austere medical care delivery system.

Logistic support

It is essential that onsite management personnel identify resupply priorities and that personnel be aware of the time of resupply and the type and amount of supplies to be expected. Although these are obvious factors, they are rarely dealt with early enough into the catastrophic event to conserve the use of critical items; thus a period of serious scarcity occurs before the care levels off.

Communications

Information from a variety of communication modes is essential if more than the most minimal austere medical care is to be given. Regardless of the communication mode used, it must be controlled and disciplined; the use of communication routes for lengthy, clever, or personal messages in this situation are therefore to be condemned.

Channels are usually scarce, and relaying medical needs may not have the highest priority if armed conflict exists or if caring for medical needs interferes with further rescue efforts. Messages must be concise and contain only information needed for decision making at higher levels, particularly at those levels that directly impact on austere medical care delivery.

Worksheet summary

Table 13-1 is a sample worksheet that can be used both for planning and training exercises and for onsite operations in an austere medical care situation.

Although it is difficult to fully anticipate the required amount of each factor for a specific situation, especially in the midst of a catastrophe, a grounding in the principles of burn and mass casualty care will enable those in charge to make a "best guesstimate" decision as to the optimum operational efficacy and austerity level of care.

In developing these worksheets and any other evaluation technique, the tendency to try to improve them always exists. Although this in itself is commendable, the improvements can make the programs more complex, and complexity isn't necessarily better. For example, adapting this type of worksheet to a computerized format (that may not be readily available in a disaster situation) defeats the basic premise for disaster planning and operational efficacy in a variety of extreme and catastrophic situations.

Table 13-1. Factors to be considered in determining the austerity level of care
to be implemented: a worksheet

Factors	Austerity level			
	I	II	III	IV
Patients				
Number				
Type				
Severity				
Evacuation time				
Personnel				
Type				
Training				
Number				
Facilities				
Shelter				
Beds				
Equipment				
Laboratory				
X-ray film				
Nonmedical				
Supplies				
Medical				
Nonmedical				
Communications				

PRINCIPLES OF AUSTERE CARE
LD_{50}

To determine the care that can be given under each of the recommended four austerity levels, it is essential to begin by determining the varying expected LD_{50}s (i.e., the estimation of survival from a baseline of 50% survival with a given percent of BSA burned). Although LD_{50} has more conventionally been used to evaluate the toxicity of substances, in the context of mass casualty care it does provide a critical point of reference in endeavoring to make best triage decisions in less than a sheltered and safe environment of a laboratory. In this perspective, LD_{50} does provide a triage guideline for those to be assigned to the expectant group in a mass casualty care situation. It is a common error to expend too many scarce resources either on this category or on the delayed category, since once the immediate lifesaving treatment is instituted, it can usually be maintained quite easily on a limited level of care, often until the crisis has subsided.

Table 13-2. Amount of second- or third-degree burn that represents LD_{50} for each austerity level

Austerity level	Degree of burn	LD_{50} (% BSA)*
0†	Second	< 90
	Third	< 70
I	Second	< 80
	Third	< 60
II	Second	< 70
	Third	< 50
III	Second	< 60
	Third	< 40
IV	Second	< 50
	Third	< 30

*Modifiers: Prognostic and/or complications: subtract 5% for each factor:
  1. Age: younger than 5 or older than 60 years of age
  2. Smoke inhalation injury
  3. Location, i.e., face, feet, hands, perineum
  4. Cardiopulmonary disease
  5. Associated major injury
†Austerity level 0: normal level of care

In Table 13-2 a comparison is presented of the LD_{50}s to be expected under the various austerity levels vs. the percent of second- and third-degree cutaneous burn. To maintain the relevancy of these data, various modifying factors need to be considered: age, smoke inhalation injury, location of injury, associated cardiopulmonary disease, and other major injuries.

Burn injury differentiations

In determining the care that can be given for each austerity level, the following burn injury differentiations should be reiterated:
  1. A major burn injury is defined as: second-degree burns of greater than 25% BSA in adults or 20% BSA in children, all third-degree burns of 10% BSA or greater, and all burns involving hands and feet.
  2. A moderate, uncomplicated burn injury is a second-degree burn of 15% to 25% BSA in adults, 10% to 20% BSA in children with less than 10% third-degree burns that do not involve eyes, ears, face, hands, feet, or perineum.
  3. A minor burn injury is a second-degree burn of less than 15% BSA in adults, 10% BSA in children, with less than 2% third-degree burn in noncritical areas.

Austere care by triage category

Discipline must again be emphasized. The care of burns in a mass casualty situation can be very demoralizing, not only to the health care workers, but to other patients and to the people at the scene of the catastrophe. This behavioral condition must be dealt with as expeditiously as possible if maximum care is to be given to all the victims and the entire rescue operation is to continue in a viable manner.

Immediate. Immediate care means performing without delay those emergency care tasks necessary to save a life or prevent further deterioration such as clearing of airway, external cardiac massage, stopping of major accessible hemorrhage, relief of pneumothorax or hemothorax, and correction of hypovolemic shock by the administration of IV fluids.

If resources permit, treatments such as the following can be extended: the use of airway or insertion of an endotracheal tube, ventilatory support either manually with an Ambu-bag, or use of various types of ventilatory support apparatus, oxygen, the correction of acid/base abnormalities, and the administration of various cardiac pharmacologic drugs.

Although much will depend on the availability of these emergency medical care resources in extreme circumstances and a likely hazardous environment, major and primary treatment pertaining to a mass casualty situation can proceed without delay. All unconscious patients have a degree of airway obstruction, relief of which can be given by minimally trained personnel by extension of the neck and mandible. This effort can be greatly assisted by use of a simple airway that could be readily available and easily inserted.

It is also presumed that all patients in shock, from whatever cause, are acidotic and will benefit from the use of Ringer's lactate solution instead of isotonic saline or plain 5% dextrose in water. The risk of overload, especially in cardiac or elderly patients and those with smoke inhalation injury, can be minimized if clinical signs are observed together with CVP readings, if available, and close monitoring of the urine output. One must be careful only to give enough fluid to maintain urinary output at minimum levels (30 to 50 ml/hour), presuming that adequate urine output reflects adequate perfusion of the kidney and other vital organs.

In an unlimited resource environment it is accepted that this corollary is not always valid, but in an austere care situation diabetes and high-output renal failure can be recognized by the simple measurement of urine specific gravity and testing for urine glucose and acetone. Unfortunately, under more extreme circumstances it may be possible to do little for these conditions, but at least continued hypovolemic shock or gross overload with subsequent congestive failure can be prevented. Cardiogenic shock may also be treatable if digitalis preparations are on hand. Obviously, the use of hypertonic saline solutions and other treatments that require frequent and sophisticated monitoring have no place in the delivery of austere medical care unless very unusual circumstances and preparations, including supplies and qualified personnel, are available. It is questionable whether improvement results with the use of these methods at any time, much less in a situation in which their use would require a massive expenditure of resources.

Similarly, both the diagnosis and treatment of pneumothorax or hemothorax can be made clinically without x-ray film equipment by physical examination and more definitively with the insertion of a needle into the pleural space and the use of a makeshift underwater seal—even without suction.

Delayed. In an austere situation the tendency exists to increase the number of patients in both this and the immediate categories. By definition, these patients are not in immediate danger of dying, yet they have injuries or diseases of such a magnitude that major treatment is essential in the long term if they are to survive.

As the austerity level becomes more severe, function or cosmesis rapidly becomes less of an issue. In treating the patients in this category, it is important to be familiar with the usual pathophysiology following severe thermal injury; i.e., the capillary permeability resulting in the development of hypovolemic shock will persist for 48 to 96 hours regardless of the treatment, and the objective during this period is to maintain perfusion of the vital organs and not to correct the hypovolemia.

Establishing an austere medical care management program at the earliest possible time that can be run by allied or paramedical personnel with only minimal supervision is essential for the effective care of the injured in this triage category.

There are several urgent austere treatment issues to recognize such as the occurrence of decreased chest wall compliance that can easily be relieved by escharotomy or that involving a survival of a limb that can be treated expeditiously with escharotomy. There is no place in austere care for early excision because of (1) the extensive demands it places on scarce personnel, and (2) most important, the marked need of blood replacement, an item otherwise not required for initial burn care.

As previously discussed, there has been and will undoubtedly continue to be a debate over crystalloid or Ringer's lactate vs. colloid solutions. The varying opinions regarding this matter emphasize at least a degree of equal efficacy of both of these treatment regimens. But, in providing austere medical care, the crystalloid solution is the only acceptable treatment for the following reasons:

1. Supplies are more readily available and more easily stored, and administration requires less skill and/or monitoring.
2. The available colloid can thus be better used in the treatment of other types of injury (e.g., hemorrhagic hypovolemic shock).

Expectant. Although the term and the category expectant explicitly refer to the fact that under the circumstances the patient is not expected to survive, some care is given. It has often been noted that patients with severe third-degree burns and hypotension are often alert and without pain. In these cases realistic comfort by nonmedically trained personnel can be most helpful.

The number of patients in this category usually increases with the extent of the mass casualty situation. Furthermore, although analgesics are given to the limit of their availability, either parenterally or even orally if need be, these patients, if hypotensive, will not absorb the medication; but they will also not be in pain.

Given the assessed irrevocable situation for patients triaged into the expectant grouping, and subject to available supplies, IV fluids and supplies should not be considered. In the event that a plentiful supply is assured, starting an IV can be helpful, if only to make health care personnel feel less helpless. Another approach is the judicious use of oral fluids, not electrolyte solutions, which can also be comforting. One of the major problems in caring for this group is the acceptance of the limited percentage of recovery by the health care personnel. In these instances, leadership, discipline, and experience are paramount.

Minimal. The treatment for this category is essentially self-care, possibly unsupervised. Yet, there is always a decision as to whether scarce or limited resources should be directed toward this group so that they may more rapidly return to function, even though by definition they will survive their burn injury, but function will not necessarily be restored. This decision depends on the situation and the value of the personnel to overall survival. If return to duty is necessary to increase the overall survival rate, the best available personnel may be directed toward their care. The use of scarce resources for this group should be strongly considered in austerity level IV and possibly in level III.

SPECIAL TREATMENT ISSUES
Resuscitation

Fortunately there are some simple expedient methods of resuscitation that can be lifesaving—such as provision of airway, ventilatory support, and external cardiac massage—and that can be readily implemented. The question is: If the resuscitation does not provide an immediate response or if there is a continuing need to expend scarce resources to prolong the patient's life, at what point should the decision be made that the care must become more austere? The ability to make this decision in a timely fashion is the basic issue of disaster burn care.

Fluid therapy

Although IV fluids only are the treatment of choice, they may be in short or high-priority supply. As a second choice in severely burned patients, oral electrolyte solutions may be used. The most commonly recommended consists of 1 teaspoonful salt and ½ teaspoonful baking soda or sodium bicarbonate in 1 quart of water every 15 minutes for 2 or 3 hours. If sufficient water is available, the total fluid intake for the first 24 hours may be estimated according to weight as 1 pint of fluid for each 20 pounds. For the second 24 hours the fluid requirements are about one half the amount estimated for the first 24 hours. After 48 hours, water and food may be taken as desired and tolerated.

For moderately burned patients, oral electrolyte solution, ½ glass, should be given every 15 minutes for 2 or 3 hours. Afterwards, 1 glass of oral electrolyte solution should be given every 4 hours for the first day; after 24 hours, ad libitum.

Wound care

The care of the burn wound in an austere situation deserves special attention. For some reason, when the usual treatments such as silver sulfadiazine and Sulfamylon are not available, there is a strong tendency to revert to antiquated home remedies instead of adopting what is available commensurate with modern concepts of burn wound care. It is important to review the principles of bacterial virulence and the relationship of quantitative bacteriology to development of burn wound sepsis. The principles of bacterial wound invasion and often adverse absorption of topical medication in both second- and third-degree burns should be considered.

The wound should be cleansed as effectively and as soon as possible after resuscitation and the commencement of stabilization procedures (1) to reduce the number, and hopefully, some of the more virulent types, of bacteria on the wound and (2) to provide a most important avenue to fully examine the wound. This procedure should be repeated twice daily, if possible. Apply no ointment, specifically no petrolatum base medications, that may seal the wound.

Only the tissue that is most easy to remove and obviously necrotic should be debrided. A gauze dressing, preferably not of the "nonadherent" type, but one that will absorb exudate, should be applied. This not only protects the wound from exposure to the elements and contaminated environments, but facilitates care and transportation. In a prolonged care situation (i.e., after the initial resuscitation period of 48 to 96 hours and if sepsis is present or imminent), use of even homemade Dakin's solution (i.e., without the buffer), simple sodium hypochlorite or bleach in a 0.25% solution, and a similar solution of acetic acid made from vinegar may be helpful. Dilute detergent of any type and abundant water are of most benefit when they are available.

Sterile technique is always desirable, but clean technique will suffice. It is vital that health care personnel cleanse their hands before they treat each new burn patient to prevent and control many of the most common infections that beset a population when public health measures break down.

Escharotomy can be lifesaving if it reduces pulmonary compliance, and it can be limb saving if a circumferential burn is compromising circulation. It should be able to be performed without blood loss.

Depending on the situation, it might be better to use the limited topical antimicrobials on the minimal patient so that they may return to function as soon as possible, since sepsis could place them in a nonfunctioning category. Their return to duty may be essential to the mission or rescue operation and/or assistance with other patients.

Prevention of sepsis and immunization

Prevention of sepsis often takes the form of clean technique; thus the amount of inoculum needed is reduced, and those with the most obvious and virulent infections are isolated. Public health measures should be stressed. A breakdown in this area, with the subsequent development of something as common as bacillary dysentery, can be fatal. The use of prophylactic antimicrobials is generally wasteful. They should be reserved for only clearly identified and easily treated infections.

The value of immunization such as for tetanus and other diseases is debatable at this point. Immunization does not replace basic public health methods such as the provision for uncontaminated water and good sewage disposal, nor does it replace sound surgical principles of debridement and wound care. In austere medical care, immunizations, like other health care resources, should be provided first to medical and/or key personnel; they should not routinely be given to those whose immunizations are current.

Table 13-3 presents illustrations of the possible treatment procedures and policies by the four triage categories for each of the four austerity levels. Although the specific treatment will vary, it is useful to introduce these procedures in management training programs in the mass casualty care domain.

It should be noted that as the austerity level becomes more severe, it is likely that medical supplies will become increasingly scarce and that the desired staffing—surgeons, physicians, nurses, or even emergency medical technicians—may not be readily available.

PLANNING FOR LOGISTIC SUPPORT

The failure to adequately plan for logistic contingencies will result in a severely diminished level of care at best, and panic at worst. Logistic contingencies translate to the provision not only of medical supplies, but also of the various general supplies for shelter, food, sanitation, energy, and communications. This is the key to the determination of the level of austerity to be practiced and the necessity to improvise, particularly as the severity level increases as a consequence of the catastrophe encountered.

Amount and type

One of the most difficult tasks in providing disaster burn care is to predict the correct amount of logistic support that will be required, not only for the burn

Table 13-3. Austerity level treatment according to triage category

Category	Treatment
Austerity level I: determinate	
Immediate	CPR, endotracheal tube ventilatory support, CVP line, indwelling catheter, ABGs, IV Ringer's lactate analgesics, no systemic antibiotics, escharotomy, wound cleansing, and topical antimicrobials
Delayed	Analgesics IV R-L, indwelling catheter, wound cleansing, and topical antimicrobials
Expectant	IM analgesics
Minimal	Wound cleansing and topical antimicrobials
Austerity level II: moderately stochastic	
Immediate	CPR, indwelling catheter, CVP, IV R-L, IM analgesics, and thoracic escharotomy
Delayed	IV R-L or oral electrolyte solution and IM analgesics
Expectant	IM or PO analgesics
Minimal	PO analgesics
Austerity level III: severely stochastic	
Immediate	CPR, IV R-L or oral electrolytes
Delayed	Oral electrolytes, PO or IM analgesics, wound cleansing, and topical antimicrobials
Expectant	IM or PO analgesics
Minimal	PO analgesics, wound cleansing, and topical antimicrobials
Austerity level IV: indeterminate	
Immediate	CPR, IV fluids, PO or IM analgesics, wound cleansing, and topical antimicrobials
Delayed	Oral fluids, PO analgesics, wound cleansing, and topical antimicrobials*
Expectant	PO analgesics
Minimal	PO analgesics, wound cleansing, and topical antimicrobials

*May elect not to expend limited topical agents at this level.

patient, but for the total medical disaster. Fortunately the supplies needed for the burn patient have become more readily available because of recent developments such as the use of crystalloid solutions, topical antimicrobials, and exposure treatment. On the other hand, in general, support requirements are increased because of open treatment modalities, and the supplies required in these situations are still substantial, especially for the delayed category.

Table 13-4 illustrates in a summary fashion the logistic support required in a mass casualty care situation (with specific reference to caring for the thermally injured) for the first three postburn days, on the basis of 100 patients per austerity level, categorized as follows: 10% immediate, 10% delayed, 10% expectant, and 70% minimal.

Benefit/cost considerations

Achieving the proper balance between the cost of purchase and stowage and the need to be prepared for an emergency requires knowledge and careful planning. Key

Table 13-4. Selected contents of a mass casualty burn kit*

Item	Austerity level			
	I	II	III	IV
Airway	20	20	20	20
Antiseptic/cleanser, topical (hexachlorophene/iodophor)	10 L	10 L	10 L	10 L
Ambu-bag	15	10	10	5
Bandage gauze 2 inches × 6 yards	150	100	100	75
Catheter, urinary, Foley (two way, No. 16)	30	20	20	10
CVP apparatus	20	20	20	10
Endotracheal/nasotracheal tube	30	20	10	5
IV tubing	50	40	30	20
Forceps, tissue	20	10	10	10
Gloves, sterile/all-purpose	250	200	150	100
Gravitometer for urinalysis	5	5	5	5
Knife handles, No. 3	20	10	10	10
Knife blades, No. 10	50	40	40	40
Knife blades, No. 20	50	40	40	40
Linen, sterile or clean	200	200	150	100
Needles, 16-gauge	50	50	50	50
Needles, 18-gauge	200	200	150	100
Needles, 21-gauge	200	200	150	100
Pads, gauze 4 inches × 48 inches	3000	2000	2000	1500
Ringer's lactate solution	300 L	250 L	250 L	200 L
Scissors, dissecting	10	10	10	10
Scissors, bandage	10	10	10	10
Silver sulfadiazine	100 kg	100 kg	100 kg	100 kg
Sulfamylon	50 kg	50 kg	50 kg	50 kg
Syringes,† 2 ml	300	200	200	150
Syringes, 20 ml	200	200	200	200
Syringes, irrigating	40	40	40	40
Thermometers	20	20	20	10
Urinalysis test tapes	300	200	200	200
Ventilatory apparatus	15	10	10	5

*Supplies required for 100 patients per austerity level.
†Since plastic cannot readily be recycled, glass syringes are desirable.

to this enigma is combining the selection of inexpensive items with long shelf life with a well-organized rotation policy. A clear understanding of the goals of austere medical care, as well as of the care needed by patients with thermal injury, is reflected in an accurate and easily accessible inventory.

Training

Like all other aspects of medical care in a disaster situation, burn care in an austere medical mode emphasizes that there is no substitute for training. It is impossible to predict, especially under a worst scenario, what role anyone may have to perform in a catastrophe involving an overwhelming number of victims. Under these circumstances it is important to recognize that nonmedical personnel may be involved at all levels of care unique to the event. Thus all aspects (e.g., terms, procedures, measurements) should be simple and common (e.g., use Fahrenheit vs. Centigrade or teaspoonful vs. milliliter).

PITFALLS AND PROBLEMS
Treatment

Most of the pitfalls and problems are not unique to mass casualty situations and reflect those described elsewhere in this text: (1) don't force the victim to eat or drink if vomiting—ileus is common; (2) don't give fluids when the person is unconscious or semiconscious; (3) don't overload—if a little urine output is good, a lot may be deadly.

Information resources

The need always arises during a disaster for further information concerning how to cope with the trauma and emergency care; how to handle public health, field sanitation, equipment repair problems, and concerning many other subjects not ordinarily referred to by medical personnel. Therefore a number of references should be set aside and kept current for austere or disaster medical practice.

Security

Although an element of unpredictability is inherent in human behavior, particularly in disaster situations, it is well accepted that people respond to authority, discipline, and leadership. However, security must be provided for, both within the facility and at the entrances. Knowledgeable individuals who also serve as guides, but not as direct health care providers, can best fulfill this often dual role.

Realistic triage

Failure to adhere to the rules by individualizing cases will lead to an unreasonable expenditure of resources, poor discipline, and diminished morale and effectiveness. If changing circumstances warrant exceptions in triage and treatment, it is far better to reappraise the austerity level decision.

Triage updates

Triaging into different categories is indicated when there is a major change in those factors directly affecting resources for immediately handling the injured. Primary indicators include updated information concerning the number of victims and their injuries and resupply and/or evacuation restrictions.

SUMMARY

Austere medical care has been identified as being straightforward, disciplined, rigorous, and often characterized as being harsh and inhumane. Yet, if understood as providing a framework within which treatment resources are most effectively allocated to the number of casualties involved, it can also be considered humane and dedicated to caring for all. Consistent with this objective, this chapter has dealt with those principles to enable health care providers both to plan and to improvise as needed in a disaster situation.

In this context, burn care in a disaster situation, like all mass casualty care, requires planning and training if optimum use is to be made of limited resources. By definition, all resources in a catastrophic situation are to be considered scarce. Therefore a level of austere medical care is always required to handle the victims involved.

Given the scarcity of resources, medical care management in this type of scenario also requires an increasing ability to improvise as the level of care possible becomes more austere. This can only be effectively accomplished with preparation, including ongoing training programs such as those under the aegis of FEMA, and with leadership in maintaining relevancy by those agencies having a mandate to handle disaster situations such as the National Disaster Medical Services (NDMS).

REFERENCES

1. Austere medical care for disaster: a reference manual for allied health workers and selected trained laymen, Public Health Service No 1071-D-1, Washington, DC, 1964, U.S. Department of Health, Education, and Welfare.
2. Baker, S, and O'Neill, B: The injury severity score: an update, J Trauma 16:882, 1976.
3. Brandt, EN, Jr, et al: Designing a national disaster medical system, Public Health Rep 100:455, 1985.
4. Champion, HR, and Sacco, WJ: Role of trauma score in triage of mass casualties, Disaster Med 1:24, 1983.
4a. Dressler, DP, Hozid, JL, and Giddon, DB: The physician and mass casualty care: a survey of Massachusetts physicians, J Trauma 11:260, 1971.
5. Enyart, JL, and Miller, DW: Treatment of burns resulting from disaster, JAMA 158:95, 1955.
5a. Giddon, DB, Fischer, TE, Dressler, DP, and Hozid, JL: Disaster preparedness for dental students, J Dent Educ 40:632, 1971.
6. Honig, A: Psychological needs of disaster workers, The Cerritos Air Disaster—The First Joint Review SCESA Conference, Los Angeles, Jan. 9, 1987. Cited by Commander W. Baker, Los Angeles Sheriff's Dept. at FEMA seminar on contemporary issues in emergency management, Emmitsburg, Md., Feb. 10, 1987.

6a. Hozid, JL, et al: An achievement test and attitude assessment in disaster preparedness for undergraduate dental students: a final report of contracts PH 110-228 and PH 110-153, January 1970.

7. Imbus, S, and Zawacki, BE: Autonomy for burned patients when survival is unprecedented, New Engl J Med 297:308, 1977.

8. Koenigsburg, FJ: Cameroon disaster and disaster worker stress. Paper presented by Col. Koenigsburg, MC USAF, Office of Foreign Disaster Assistance, Agency for International Development, Washington, DC, at the FEMA seminar on contemporary issues in emergency management, Emmitsburg, Md., Feb. 10, 1987.

9. Orr, GE: Combat operations C3I: fundamentals and interactions, Maxwell Air Force Base, Alabama, 1983, Air University Press.

9a. Parad, HJ, Resnick, HLP, and Parad, LG, editors: Emergency and disaster management: a mental health sourcebook, Bowie, MD, 1976, The Charles Press Publishers, Inc.

10. Quarentelli, EL: Delivery of emergency medical services in disaster: assumptions and realities, New York, 1983, Irvington Publisher, Inc.

11. Rozin, RR: Integration of military unit and civilian hospital during mass casualty situation: experience during the 1982 Lebanon war, Milit Med 151:580, 1986.

12. Shaftan, GW: Disaster and medical care, J Trauma 2:111, 1962.

13. Sutherland, JW: Systems: analysis, administration, and architecture, New York, 1981, Van Nostrand Reinhold Co, Inc.

14. Walters, CW, and Phillips, AW: Mass burns. Proceedings of a workshop, 12-14 March 1968, Washington, DC: National Academy of Sciences, Pub No NTIS, AD-689-495: PC A18, Springfield, VA, 1969, US Dept of Commerce.

15. Zawacki, BE: Clinical, legal and moral perspectives, J Trauma 21:695, 1981.

Index